Mona Rabea is a phoniatrician with MSc of Phoniatrics (2017), M.B.B.Ch. (2008), Faculty of Medicine, Mansoura University, Egypt. She is interested in academic writing on phoniatrics.

This book is dedicated to the soul of my father who always pushed me forward (I hope for him the highest degrees in the paradise), my mother who is more than an angel, my supportive husband, my two little flowers (Malak and Mawadda), all my inspiring family members and to those who loved me without restriction.

Mona Rabea

PHONOLOGICAL ERROR PATTERNS FROM A CLINICAL PERSPECTIVE

AUSTIN MACAULEY PUBLISHERS™

LONDON • CAMBRIDGE • NEW YORK • SHARJAH

ISBN – 9789948258452 – (Paperback)
ISBN – 9789948258445 – (E-Book)

Application Number: MC-10-01-2025727
Age Classification: E

First Published (2021)
AUSTIN MACAULEY PUBLISHERS FZE
Sharjah Publishing City
P.O Box [519201]
Sharjah, UAE
www.austinmacauley.ae
+971 655 95 202

Firstly, I want to thank Almighty Allah for everything. We can never thank Allah enough for the continuous grace, mercy and guidance that fill our lives. Then I want to thank all my teachers and professors in all the stages of my life who always encouraged me.

Table of Contents

List of Figures

List of Tables

Preface

This book is a book on clinical phonology aiming to provide a clinical view of phonological error patterns to simplify the diagnosis of speech sound disorders for phoniatricians and speech-language pathologists. Indeed, before talking about phonological error patterns, firstly, readers should be familiar with the dual nature of speech (phonology and articulation) and the normal speech development, thus Chapter 1 discusses the difference between phonology and articulation. Chapter 2 describes the normal speech development and its theories, Chapter 3 is an overview of phonological error patterns reaching Chapter 4 which describes the approach to diagnosis of speech sound disorders.

In my first work with phonological error patterns for my master thesis's research, I found it hard to understand and interpret phonology, may be because it was the first time to interact with this information, as I am a physician who studied the medical view of human body not the linguistic view of his brain. Later on, after a lot of readings and applying the known information on many cases, I reached an easy practical view of diagnosis of speech sound disorders hoping to deliver this information to my colleagues in this interesting field and help the unintelligible children to be easily diagnosed and treated to communicate freely with their words.

My experience with phonological error patterns taught me that the Almighty Allah has created everything within a system, even the misarticulations of children during acquisition of their speech are systematic and have normal physiology to reach certain milestones. A deviation from that, indicates that the child has a disorder and is need of treatment.

Simply, language including its four domains (semantics, grammar (morphology, syntax), phonology and pragmatics) is like any organ in the body and has a normal path (physiology) in its learning.

When the child acquires phonology, he makes errors during his attempt to imitate adult's words like his attempts during learning his first steps of walking. As he grows, he tries to modify and suppress these errors until reach adults' form. These error patterns have certain path with each age interval. Children with phonological disorders which comprise the main group of speech sound disorders use different path from normal; as they may use error patterns rarely used by the normal children (unusual error patterns); they may persist to use the normal error patterns after the age of their suppression (delayed error patterns); and they may also apply the normal error patterns across multiple contexts than normal (gross included error patterns). Thus, the gold standards for diagnosis of phonological disorders in any language is the knowledge of age-appropriate error patterns, their ages of suppression and their appropriate inclusion in each age interval and the unusual error patterns in that language.

Children with phonological disorders are often presented with unintelligibility. Some clinicians do not know how to start. Simply, at first, the child's word consistency should be assessed to know if he is consistent in using his words or not, if the child is consistent, he should have phonological error patterns assessment to identify the types of his error patterns. When the child has just a phonological delay, he uses delayed error patterns, but when he uses unusual error patterns alone or with other types of phonological error patterns, he may have a consistent atypical phonological disorder. On the other side, inconsistent child may have inconsistent phonological disorder or childhood apraxia of speech that should be differentiated by its type criteria. Also, articulation abilities of the child should be also assessed to identify phonetic errors and decide if it matched with his age or not and if it's stimulable or not. Thus, bimodal assessment of speech (i.e. phonological and articulation models) is a systematic one.

Intelligibility should be assessed to determine the child's age of intelligibility and factors affecting it like prosody. Also, severity should be assessed; for articulation errors by percent of consonant and vowels correct and for phonological error patterns by phonological error patterns density index to determine degree of severity and monitor improvement after therapy.

In this book, I preview the information of phonological error patterns and speech sound disorders in a new way like I have learned in the faculty of medicine which firstly presents the normal physiology then the meaning of the disorder and how to reach its diagnosis. Hoping to enjoy reading and get benefits.

Chapter 1:
Difference Between
Phonology and Articulation

Chapter Outlines

o Dual nature of speech.
o Difference between phonology and articulation.
o How to differentiate phonological disorders from articulation disorders?

Humans are given a magnificent communicative ability. You can imagine that with a limited set of sounds, a speaker of any language can express an unlimited number of sentences. These human speech sounds have no meaning in themselves, but become meaningful when combined with each other and controlled with certain linguistic systems. For instance, /s/, /t/ and /m/ lack meaning when set alone, however, when enrolled by English language system, they make words such as (sun, it, me and myth) (Bleile, 2014). Communication disorder can be defined as a disability to understand or express meaning between partners. Developmental disorders of communication represent one of the most common reasons for paediatric referrals (Harel et al., 1996). Most children who are referred for clinical assessment of a communication disorder have a speech disorder. Their speech is unintelligible because it is characterised by many mispronunciations of words (Dodd, 2013).

Dual Nature of Speech:

Speech is important because of its dual nature in communication, being an aspect of language and a mode of expression. The dual nature of speech is the basis of the conceptual difference between phonology (a perception, knowledge or linguistic aspect) and articulation (a production, motor or phonetic aspect) (figure 1) (Bleile, 2014).

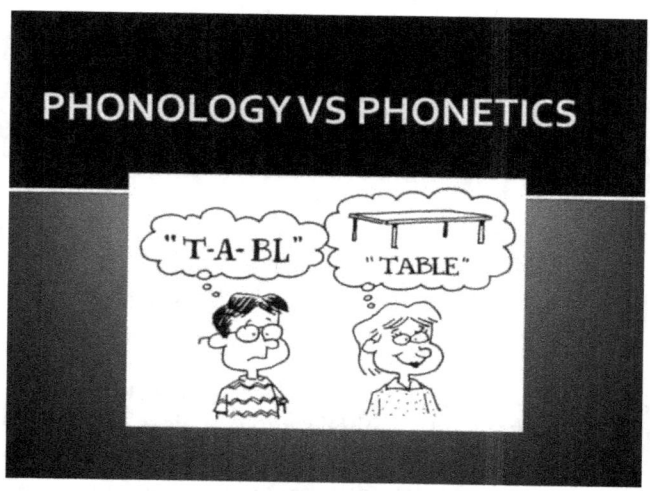

Figure 1: Difference Between Phonology and Phonetics (Articulation)

(Source: http://www.differencebetween.info/)

Difference between Phonology and Articulation:

Phonology is the study of the speech sound system of a language or the smallest unit of language that overlays meaning onto the motor movements of speech (Shulman and Singleton, 2013). Thus, it is considered a major component of language (figure 2, 3), along with morphology (word form), syntax (word order), semantics (word meaning) and pragmatics (social usage) (Gordon-Brannan et al, 2007).

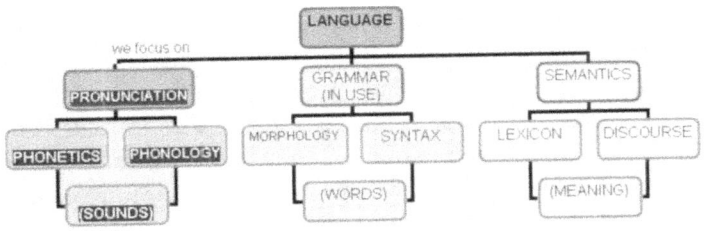

Figure 2: Components of Spoken Language

(source: http://alejandronunez-a-3.blogspot.com/p/auditory-phonetics.html)

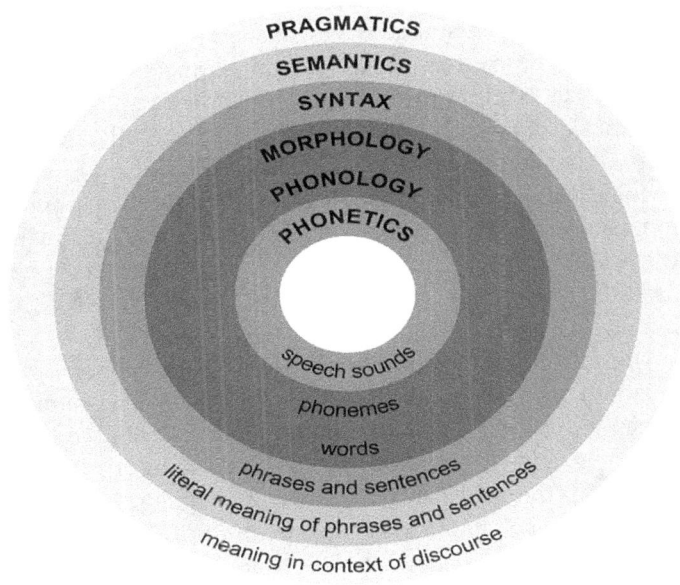

Figure 3: Levels of Spoken Language
(various parts of language and their meanings are shown by this figure)

(Source: https://courses.lumenlearning.com/boundless-psychology/chapter/introduction-to-language/)

Phonology means the formulation of sound sequences based on knowledge of the phonological system of a language that comprises phonemic inventory (phonemes) representing various classes (based on distinctive physiological and acoustic characteristic) and a set of phonotactic rules (how these phonemes can be arranged in syllables to form words) (Gordon-Brannan et al, 2007). Simply, it's the study of a set of phonemes which make up a certain language and how they are combined, organised and structured into syllables, morphemes and words (Barrett, 2016).

Acquisition of phonology depends on the cognitive abilities that allow children to identify phonemes and realise the phonotactic rules of a language they are learning to speak (Kuhl, 2004). During this period of development, children make many speech sound errors that are often patterned or systematic. These errors are called phonological error patterns and applied to phonemic classes rather than to individual phonemes, e.g. some children systematically replace fricatives in adult target words with stops (Geirut et al., 1996). Phonological error patterns do not only affect a group of phonemes shared in a common dimension, but may also affect the syllable structure of the word, sound sequences like a cluster, so that, phonological error patterns can affect any phonological element classes.

The developing child tends to use the phonological opposition member that puts the least strain on a human's speech ability, e.g. children merge the potential contrast between /t/ and /k/, resulting in production of [t], the easy member of the pair. A child whose language requires a contrast between /t/ and /k/ will learn from experience to suppress this error pattern (velar fronting) and produce the contrast between /t/ and /k/ (Miccio & Scarpino, 2009). Therefore, a natural phonological error pattern is generally said to be phonetically motivated due to perceptual, articulatory, or acoustic factors and to involve the simplification of a more complex articulation (Bernhardt and Stoel-Gammon, 1997), e.g. stopping where the reverse would not occur naturally because fricatives have the more difficult property (Miccio and Scarpino, 2009).

In contrast to phonology, which is concerned with perception and knowledge, Articulation depends on motor systems for planning, programming and execution of complex sequences of rapid, fine movements using muscles of the vocal tract integrating air flow to produce speech sounds (Dodd et al., 2018). Thus, the articulation is referred to as the phonetic or mechanical part of speech. It comprises the speech sounds that are produced (articulatory), heard (acoustics) and perceived (auditory) as the result of movements of the articulators.

How to Differentiate Phonological Disorders from Articulation Disorders?

Differentiating between phonological error patterns and articulation errors (table 1) is very important, as each error type has its clinical implications for diagnosis and treatment. Clinicians may find it difficult, however, it can be differentiated as the following: errors affecting the syllable structure of the word are phonological error patterns, while substitutions errors (replacing one phoneme with another one) have some debates, they may be; assimilation error patterns; substitution error patterns; or articulation substitution errors. In assimilation error patterns, a similar phoneme is found in the word. On the other hand, substitution error patterns, there is no similar phoneme in the word and errors are stimulable for most age-appropriate speech sounds and child's articulation is not affected (Dodd et al., 2013).

In contrast to substitution error patterns, a child with an articulation substitution error is unable to articulate a perceptually acceptable production of the affected sounds, in isolation, syllables and words or in any phonetic context, misarticulating these sounds in the same way at every attempt (Dodd, 2014). However, to decide that child's misarticulation is due to an articulation disorder and not a normal developmental misarticulation of these sounds (i.e. the sound not present in the phonetic inventory yet), Clinicians should use the developmental acquisition chart of speech sounds of the child's language to be a reference for normative data (i.e. the child should past the age of a certain sound acquisition to be affected).

Another point of difference is that phonological error patterns usually occur in specific phonetic contexts, so that, a speech sound may be correct in some contexts, but not in others; while articulation errors are consistent errors occurring in all contexts (Dodd et al., 2018). Sometimes, the child may make inconsistent articulation error of certain speech sound pasting the normal age of acquisition of that sound, occurring for example, in one or two positions of the word only, that means that the child is acquiring that sound but not generalised in all phonetic contexts yet and that sound needs to be remediated in the affected contexts only.

Table 1: Articulation Disorders Versus Phonological Disorders *(Bauman-Waengler, 2008)*

Phonological Disorders	Articulation Disorders
Linguistically based (i.e. no difficulty in executing movements for speech, but difficulties are in understanding the rules of language).	Motor based (i.e. Difficulty in producing movements for speech).
Knowledge errors	Surface errors
Phonemic errors	Phonetic errors
Stimulable errors	Non-stimulable errors
Occur in specific phonetic contexts	Occur in all phonetic contexts
Impacts other areas of language (morphology, syntax, semantics and pragmatics).	Does not impact other areas of language.

Chapter Summary

This chapter describes the two aspects of speech where phonology is the knowledge of certain language phonemes and how they are organised to form words; while articulation is the planning, programming and execution of motor movements of articulators to pronounce words. Ways to differentiate phonological disorders from articulation disorders are also described.

References

Barrett, M. (2016). The development of language. Psychology Press.

Bauman-Waengler, J. (2008): Articulatory and phonological impairments: A clinical focus (3rd Ed.). Boston: Allyn and Bacon.

Bernhardt, B., & Stoel-Gammon, C. (1997). Grounded phonology: Application to the analysis of disordered speech. The New Phonologies: developments in clinical linguistics, 163-210.

Bleile, K. M. (2014). The manual of speech sound disorders: A book for students and clinicians. Cengage Learning.

Capone Singleton, N., & Shulman, B. (2013). Language development: Foundations, processes, and clinical applications. Burlington, MA: Jones & Bartlett Publishers.

Carson, C., Klee, T., Carson D., & Hime, L. (2003). Phonological profiles of, 28-29.

Dodd, B. (2013). Differential diagnosis and treatment of children with speech disorder. John Wiley & Sons.

Dodd, B. (2014). Differential diagnosis of pediatric speech sound disorder. Current Developmental Disorders Reports, 1(3), 189-196.

Dodd, B., Reilly, S., Ttofari Eecen, K., & Morgan, A. T. (2018). Articulation or phonology? Evidence from longitudinal error data. Clinical linguistics & phonetics, 32(11), 1027-1041.

Gierut, J. A., Morrisette, M. L., Hughes, M. T., & Rowland, S. (1996). Phonological treatment efficacy and developmental norms. Language, Speech, and Hearing Services in Schools, 27(3), 215-230.

Gordon-Brannan, M. E., & Weiss, C. E. (2007). Clinical management of articulatory and phonologic disorders. Lippincott Williams & Wilkins.

Harel, S., Greenstein, Y., Kramer, U., Yifat, R., Samuel, E., Nevo, Y., & Shinnar, S. (1996). Clinical characteristics of children referred to a child development center for evaluation of speech, language, and communication disorders. Pediatric neurology, 15(4), 305-311.

Kuhl, P. K. (2004). Early language acquisition: cracking the speech code. Nature reviews neuroscience, 5(11), 831.

Miccio, A. W., & Scarpino, S. E. (2009). 25 Phonological Analysis, Phonological Processes. The handbook of clinical linguistics, 412.

Shulman, B. B., & Singleton, N. C. (2013). Language Development: Foundations, Processes, and Clinical Applications. Jones & Bartlett Publishers.

Waring, R., Eadie, P., Rickard Liow, S., & Dodd, B. (2018). The phonological memory profile of preschool children who make atypical speech sound errors. Clinical linguistics & phonetics, 32(1), 28-45.

Chapter 2:
Speech Development and Theories of Acquisition

Chapter Outlines

Stages of Speech Development

Acquiring adult-like speech is a year-long process that starts as early as language development itself and is reasonably well established by the age of 4 or 5 years. Appropriate lexical input, acquisition of a stable phonological system and fine coordination of articulators are required to reach adult-like speech (Neves et al., 1999). Generally, speech development has been described by Gordon-Brannan and Weiss (2007) as series of six stages:

Stage 1: Prelinguistic Stage (0-1 Year):

Children communicate through crying and gestures (reflexive vocalisations). During the end of this period speech-like vocalisations or babbling predominate.

Stage 2: First Words (1-1½ Years):

Meaningful speech production emerges ending with an expressive vocabulary of about 50 words. The syllable structure of these words is characterised by being simple, such as CV, CVC and CVCV. Consonants produced are primarily stops, nasals and glides. The words seem to be produced as whole units rather than as words composed of individual phonemes.

Stage 3: Phonemic Development (1½-4 Years)

This is the phonological stage of single morphemes. During this stage, word productions are no longer whole-word units, but rather are composed of phonemes. Phonetic inventory is increased and misarticulations of most speech sounds nearly disappear by 4 years of age. The number of different sound classes, phonemes and syllable structures increases and phonological elements become more complex with adding consonant clusters and multisyllabic words to the linguistic component of speech. During this period, many children use phonological error patterns, however, the child gradually discontinues applying phonological error patterns and the normally developing 4-year-old child produces most phonemic contrasts correctly at least some of the time.

Stage 4: Stabilisation of the Phonological System (4-8 Years)

Children complete acquisition of the adult system as reflected by stabilisation of the production of the speech sounds that were variably produced and acquisition of the remaining sounds. They learn the production of all troublesome sounds by age of 7 years. Additionally, they gain more understanding of the phonemic system as they begin to read and write.

Stage 5: Morphophonemic Development (7-12 Years)

Phonological development continues as they acquire morphophonemic rules and a more elaborate derivational structure of the language. Children learn how to spell and read, use vowel shifts and apply contrastive stress for differentiating compound words from noun phrases such as *blackboard* from *black board*. Morphophonemic alterations are learned, such as changes between *electric* and *electricity* in which the final /k/ in *electric* becomes /s/ in *electricity*. Thus, phonological acquisition is not complete by age 7 years as has been traditionally thought. It continues until 12 years of age and perhaps even longer when mastery of spelling is considered. However, sound production of the approximately 50 sounds in the English language usually is mastered by 7 years of age.

Stage 6: Spelling (12-+16 Years):

During this stage, spelling skills are acquired and perfected.

Prerequisites for Normal Phonemic and Phonetic Development:

Speech development can be analysed in two ways: phonemic versus phonetic development. Knowledge of the prerequisites for the normal phonemic and phonetic aspects of speech development facilities identification of the cause of phonological or articulation disorder.

- ***Prerequisites for Normal Phonemic Development (Stoel-Gammon, 2001):***
1. Intact sensory system (hearing and vision).
2. Sufficient linguistic input.
3. Appropriate cognitive abilities enough to perceive store and retrieve phonological representations.

- ***Taxonomy of Phonological Acquisition (Ingram and Ingram, 2001):***

Children differ in their course of phonological acquisition. Therefore, they are classified into the following types:

1. *The phonologically precocious child:* The child's phonological system is in advance of his language development; his speech is characterised by unexpected high intelligibility.
2. *The typically developing child:* The child's phonological system is consistent with what would be

33

expected for his language development (i.e. age-appropriate). Age-appropriate phonological error patterns are defined by Dodd et al. (2003) as error patterns used by more than 10% of the children in the same age range.

3. *The phonologically disordered child:* The child's phonological system is behind his language development; the greater the discrepancy, the greater the perception of impairment. His phonological system may be characterised by one or more of the following properties:

a. *Delayed patterns:* The child may show error patterns that are consistent with those found in younger children. Delayed phonological error patterns are normal error patterns used by less than 10% of the children in the same age range where 90% of children do not use these errors.

b. *Gross inclusion*: Error patterns may be normal, but they extend across a greater range of contexts than found in his peers.

c. *Unusual patterns:* The child may demonstrate one or more unusual error patterns. Unusual error patterns are defined by Dodd et al. (2003) as error patterns used by less than 10% of children of any age range interval.

- *Prerequisites for Normal Phonetic Development (Gordon-Brannan and Weiss, 2007):*
1. Normal anatomy and physiology of the vocal tract.
2. Intact innervation of muscles of the vocal tract.
3. Normal sensory feedback, including tactile, kinaesthetic and auditory.
4. Good motivation with presence of sufficient opportunities for articulation and reinforcement.

- *Taxonomy of Phonetic Acquisition (Amayreh and Dyson, 1998):*

34

Concerning phonetic acquisition, there are three types of age of acquisition:

1. Age of customary production: At least 50% of children in an age group produce the sound correctly in at least two-word positions.
2. Age of acquisition: At least 75% of children in an age group produce the sound correctly in all positions.
3. Age of mastery: At least 90% of children in an age group produce the sound correctly in all positions.

Phonological Acquisition Theories (Gordon-Brannan and Weiss, 2007):

No current theory is completely adequate enough to explain phonological development, although each theory does account for some required aspects. Generally, there are six major phonological acquisition theories with variations on the theme of each type of them.

A-Generative Phonology Theory:

Chomsky and Halle (1968) posited that there is an explicit set of distinctive features from which phonemes are generated. The underlying representation of a phoneme is its distinctive features. In this theory, phonological rules are applied to the underlying representations to form the surface representations, a process called 'derivation'. Phonological rules connect the knowledge component with the production component of a language to derive surface.

B-Structuralist Theory:

Jakobson (1968) emphasised that universals exist in the acquisition of language in which the phonological development and systems of all languages are similar. They also contend that an invariant and innate order of stages of phonemic development in the learning of all languages exists, however, the rate of progression through the stages of development is individual and variable.

C-Behaviourist Theory:

Olmstead (1971) emphasised the role of reinforcement in speech acquisition. It necessitates the occurrence of imitating, practising, experiencing, conditioning and reinforcing behaviour.

D-Natural Phonology Theory:

Stampe (1979) announced that the child starts with a group of innate simplification phonological error patterns which he uses to approximate adult speech. As his perception of the adult system and his production capabilities improve, he gradually eliminates these processes one by one via suppression, limitation and ordering until his speech resembles the adult's. Some segments, sound classes, consonant and vowel systems, types of syllables, rules and patterns are more natural than others. The more natural ones are those that are learned sooner by children and that appear in more languages. Examples for the most common or natural vowel system is /i.a.u/, the most natural stop system is /p.t.k/ and the most common syllable type is CV (consonant/vowel) (Edwards and Shriberg, 1983).

E-Optimality Theory:

McCarthy and Prince (1993) posited that input (underlying representations) and output representations (surface structure) exist and constraints generate surface (output) representations, not rules. A constraint is defined as "a limit on what constitutes a possible pronunciation of a word", some constraints are more important than others and thus are ranked higher and others are not as important and sometimes can be ignored. This ranking differs in different languages and in different children.

F-Nonlinear Phonology Theory:

According to Bernhardt and Stoel-Gammon (1994), in the nonlinear approach, segments composed of features are organised hierarchically rather than as bundles of features. In this approach to describe phonological acquisition, separate levels of representation or tiers for various prosodic and segmental units are organised hierarchically (i.e. word, foot, syllable, onset-rime, skeletal and segmental (phoneme) tiers.

Chapter Summary

This chapter describes the normal stages of speech development and the normal prerequisites for phonemic and phonetic acquisition which facilitates later on identification of the cause of articulation and phonological disorders. Children are classified as phonologically precocious, typically developing and phonologically disordered children according to their level in the course of acquisition. Phonological acquisition theories are also described.

References

Amayreh, M. M., & Dyson, A. T. (1998). The acquisition of Arabic consonants. Journal of Speech, Language, and Hearing Research, 41(3), 642-653.

Bernhardt, B. H, and Stoel-Gammon, C. (1994): Nonlinear Phonology Introduction and Clinical Application. Journal of Speech, Language, and Hearing Research, 37(1), 123-143.

Castro, S. L., Neves, S., Gomes, I., & Vicente, S. (1999). The development of articulation in European Portuguese: A cross-sectional study of 3-to 5-years-olds naming pictures. In Proceedings of the 5th International Congress of the International Society of Applied Psycholinguistics. Porto.

Chomsky, N., and Halle, M. (1968). The sound pattern of English. A book published by Harper and Row, inc., New York, USA.

Edwards, M. L., and Shriberg, L. D. (1983): Phonology: Applications in communicative disorders. College Hill Press.

Gordon-Brannan, M. E., & Weiss, C. E. (2007). Clinical management of articulatory and phonologic disorders. Lippincott Williams & Wilkins.

Ingram, D., and Ingram, K. D. (2001): A whole-word approach to phonological analysis and intervention. Language, speech, and hearing services in schools, 32(4), 271-283.

Jakobson, R. (1968). Child language: aphasia and phonological universals (No. 72). Walter de Gruyter.

McCarthy, J. J., and Prince, A. (1993): Generalized alignment Linguistics Department Faculty Publication Series. 12. (pp. 79-153). Springer Netherlands.

Olmsted, D. L. (1971). Out of the Mouth of Babes: Earliest Stages in Language Learning (Janua Linguarum Series Minor 117).

Stampe, D. (1979). Dissertation on natural phonology (Vol. 22). Taylor & Francis.

Stoel-Gammon, C. (2001). Down syndrome phonology: Developmental patterns and intervention strategies.

Chapter 3:
Overview of Phonological
Error Patterns

Chapter Outlines

o Definition.
o Identification criteria for phonological error patterns.
o Classification of phonological error patterns.
o Age of suppression of phonological error patterns.
o Methods of assessment of phonological error patterns.
o Selection criteria for target words used in assessment of phonological error patterns.
o Phonetic transcription and analysis method.

Definition

Bauman-Waengler (2004) defined phonological error patterns as systematic changes in sound classes, sound sequences or syllable structure.

Identification Criteria for Phonological Error Patterns

Phonologists differ in the determination of the identification criteria of phonological error patterns. The existence of a particular error pattern by single occurrence of an error is questionable. An error pattern is a general tendency that affects a group of phonological elements. A distinction should be made between one instance of an error, which may take place by chance or occur due to developmental fluctuation and the frequent occurrence of a type of error that represents a certain tendency in a child's phonological system (Dodd et al., 2003). Roberts et al. (1990) considered only one occurrence of the error pattern as evidence that the pattern is used by children. For example, if a child omitted /k/ in /make/, the production was listed under the error pattern of final consonant deletion (FCD). Other examples of omission of final /k/ or consonants in a variety of words were not required to list FCD as an error pattern in the child's phonological system.

McReynolds and Elbert (1981) suggested that for validating the presence of error pattern, specific errors have to occur in at least four examples and the error has to occur in at least 20% of the opportunities that could be affected by the error pattern. McReynolds and Elbert (1981) explained "if the child's sample contained 20 words with final consonants, at least four of the 20 words (20%) had to be produced without a final consonant to list FCD as an error pattern present in the child's phonological system." However, Kirk and Vigeland (2015) stated that this cut-off is probably too low for some types of errors which have the potential to affect a large number of phonemes such as cluster reduction (CR).

Hodson and Paden (1991) suggested that a specific error pattern must have at least 40% occurrence before being selected as a phonological error pattern. Error patterns that occur in less than 40% of opportunities would be monitored but not addressed in therapy. Similarly, Lowe (1996) suggested that the minimal requirements for qualifying a sound change as a phonological error pattern are that the error must affect more than one sound from a given sound class and the sound change must occur in at least 40% of the time. Dodd et al. (2003) used a minimum of five occurrences of a phonological error pattern in each child's large representative speech sample for establishing norms.

Whatever, there is currently no sufficient research indicating what constitutes a sufficient number of opportunities for concluding that a child's phonological system displays a particular phonological error pattern, however, most phonologists assured that the smallest grouping possible would have two members that share some dimension. Thus, the phonological change has to occur twice to qualify as a phonological error pattern for classification.

But for therapy, it depends on the sort of assessment of an error pattern, if clinicians use spontaneous sample speech, the error pattern should occur 40% of the analysed words to qualify the error pattern as active one needing remediation. When normalised testes for error pattern is available, it is easy for clinicians to compare number of child's errors with the normative data of his peers in the same age interval.

Classification of Phonological Error Patterns

The phonological error patterns that commonly occur during normal language development are called normal error patterns. Error patterns that have never been documented in normal children or that occur infrequently in the normal children are called unusual error patterns (Gammon and Dunn, 1985). Even though there are different classification systems for phonological error patterns, the focus should be on identifying them in order to reduce their existence (Bosch, 2004). Gordon-Brannan and Weiss (2007) consolidates several classification systems and divides phonological error patterns into four categories: (1) syllable structure, (2) assimilation or harmony, (3) feature contrast or substitution and (4) others (unusual error patterns and articulatory shifts).

1-Word and Syllable-Level Error Patterns:

These error patterns affect the syllabic shape of a word (Miccio and Scarpino, 2009). They change the consonant/vowel (CV) makeup of the syllables of standard adult word forms. The modifications tend to go toward a CV construction by changing number and/or sequence of vowels and consonants in the target word. These error patterns are most frequently seen in younger children with mean length of utterances between one and four morphemes (Prater and Swift, 1982). The most common syllable structure error patterns are syllable deletion, cluster reduction and final consonant deletion.

I – Syllable Deletion:

Syllable deletion, sometimes referred to as syllable omission or syllable reduction occurs when one or more syllables of a multisyllabic word is deleted. A subtype is unstressed syllable deletion or weak syllable deletion (WSD) that describes omission of an unstressed syllable in a multisyllabic word, usually the weak syllable before a strong syllable, e.g. 'potato'→ [teto], 'banana' → [nænæ] (Miccio and Scarpino, 2009).

WSD usually affects non-final weak syllables (NFWS) rather than final weak syllables (FWS). NFWS are the initial weak syllables such as 'giraffe' and the within-word weak syllables (WWWS) such as in 'telephone'. WSD occurs in normally and abnormally developing speech. Its use is affected by the numbers of syllables in words and the serial position of the weak syllable in words. Patterns of WSD use in abnormally developing speech may differ to that in normally developing as children with Specific Language Impairment (SLI) deletes more WWWS and fewer IWS than typically developing children (Carter and Gerken, 2003). Most phonologists use the term "weak syllable deletion" only without dealing with the other aspects of syllable deletion. Thus, patterns of syllable deletion should be analysed as either stressed SD or unstressed SD, non-final or final SD, one or multi SD and syllable shape (e.g. cv, cvc or cvcc) SD to provide more data about normal patterns of SD occurring in normally developing speech and unusual patterns of SD that occur in abnormally developing speech.

II – Final Consonant Deletion:

The error pattern of FCD occurs when the syllable coda in the target word is deleted (Kirk and Vigeland, 2015). Dyson and Paden (1983) defined FCD as deletion of a postvocalic singleton consonant or entire postvocalic cluster so the final form of the word ends with a vowel, e.g. 'gate' →[ge], 'most'→ [mo]. It is common in children between the ages of 1½ and 3 years, but are rare beyond three years of age (Ingram, 1989). However, the deletion of word-final clusters should not be classified as FCD, if that deletion is specific to clusters. For example, a child who produces the final consonant in 'bus' and 'cake' but deletes the entire cluster in 'desk' displays the error pattern of cluster deletion, not FCD. This child has the ability to produce singleton coda consonants but is not able to produce all cluster types in syllable codas. Similarly, the deletion of the final consonant in a consonant cluster (e.g. 'hand'→ [hær]) should not be classified as FCD but instead as cluster reduction. This is supported by the fact that most children who produce 'hand' as [hæn] do not have difficulty producing the final consonant in 'bed' (Schneider et al., 2004). A child who deletes the final singleton or cluster needs audiological evaluation as most hearing-impaired children delete the final consonant.

III – Cluster Reduction:

Gordon-Brannan and Weiss (2007) defined a cluster as two or more abutting consonants, regardless of whether the consonants appear in the same syllable or in two different syllables. However, other phonologists (e.g. Bankson and Bernthal, 1990; Hodson and Paden, 1991) describe the cluster as two contiguous consonants in the same syllable and that definition seems to be more suitable as each syllable can be produced with different breath, so that the blends should be in the same syllable.

Cluster reduction can be divided into three subcategories (Kirk and Vigeland, 2015):

A-Cluster deletion (Total Cluster Reduction).

When all consonants in a cluster are deleted (deletion of an entire cluster), the deviation may be labelled cluster deletion, e.g. 'stop' → [op]. It is the earliest occurring cluster errors and occurs only rarely in the speech of young children.

B-Cluster reduction (Partial Cluster Reduction):

In the second stage of cluster development, children reduce target words containing two consonants in the syllable onset or syllable coda to a single consonant. They may also reduce target clusters with three consonants either to two consonants or to a single consonant, e.g. 'snake' →[neɪk] and 'splash' →[blæʃ] or [bæʃ]. The deleted consonant can be an obstruent or a sonorant, e.g. [tet] for 'skate' and [bek] for 'break'.

Cluster reduction occur with certain tendency to affect certain phonemic classes and this may be related to the developing phonological abilities of the children by deleting the weaker phonemes to simplify and facilities target word's pronunciation. Thus, the most common reduction patterns are described as (Bloch, 2011):

- In *(stop + liquid)* cluster, the stop is usually maintained and the liquid deleted, e.g. 'blue'→ [bu], 'bread'→ [bed].
- In postvocalic cluster composed of *(liquid + stop)* or *(liquid + nasal)*, the liquid is usually deleted, e.g. 'bark'→ [bɑk].
- In *(s+ stop and s+ nasal)* cluster, /s/ is usually deleted, e.g. 'skip'→ [kip], 'snow'→ [no].

As children become older, the occurrence of cluster reduction diminishes (Roberts et al., 1990). Consonant clusters are typically mastered after the age of three years (Smit, 1993). Thus, cluster reduction is one of the last phonological error patterns to disappear in the speech of normal children and it is one of the most common difficulties for children with a speech sound disorders (McLeod et al., 1997).

C-Cluster substitution:
The third stage in cluster development is cluster substitution. This error pattern occurs when the correct number of consonants are produced, but one or more consonants are replaced by a different consonant (Kirk and Vigeland, 2015). At this stage of cluster development, a common error pattern is the insertion of schwa between two consonants in a cluster, e.g. 'slide' → as [sə'laɪd] (Smit,

1993). Kirk and Vigeland (2015) suggested that errors involving cluster substitution and vowel epenthesis are more advanced stages in the development of clusters than the error pattern of cluster reduction.

IV – Coalescence:

Coalescence has been described in two different ways: the first type is *coalescence of cluster* and is considered a form of cluster reduction, this deviation has been characterised as the replacement of two consonants with a different consonant that contains phonetic features of the two target consonants of a cluster, e.g. 'smoke'→ [fok] in which /f/ has the stridency feature of /s/ and the labialness of /m/ (Hodson, 2004). The second type is *coalescence of syllables* and considered a form of syllable deletion, as it is applied to syllables of multisyllabic words such that a speaker produces a multisyllabic word with fewer syllables than the underlying form with segments from both syllables being retained e.g. 'melon' → [men] for which contains /me./ from the first syllable and /n/ from the second syllable. Both types of coalescence result in a change in the structure of the syllable.

V – Epenthesis:

Gordon-Brannan and Weiss (2007) referred to Epenthesis as the addition of a phoneme to a word. The addition is often a vowel, often /ə/, although consonants are sometimes added as well. Added vowels commonly occur between two consonants of a consonant cluster and after a final voiced stop. An example of the first case is [bəlæk] for 'black' and of the second case. [mʌdə] for 'mud'. An example of adding a consonant is [fwʌn] for 'fun'. Another classification should be used for epenthesis, it may be syllabic or phonemic (adding either vowel or consonant). Although adding vowel may be considered as developing stage in the development of clusters, adding a new syllable to the word or consonant to form a cluster generally are unusual patterns.

VI – Diminutisation:

Diminutisation is adding /i/ or /I/or consonant plus /i/ to the end of a word. The resulting word is considered an immature speech pattern ("baby talk") and typically occurs during the first 50-word stage of language development. This pattern is also a form of epenthesis, e.g. 'hat' → [hæti].

VII – Doubling:

Doubling is repeating a word, usually a monosyllabic word, resulting in a multisyllabic word, e.g. 'bad'→ [bæbæ]. This deviation is also a form of epenthesis. Although different, this deviation is similar to the error pattern of reduplication, which can occur in multisyllabic words and is categorised as a harmony or assimilation error pattern.

2-Assimilation Error Patterns:

Assimilation error patterns may occur due to certain property possessed by certain segments, sometimes only in certain types of morphemes; such segments exert a triggering influence initiating assimilation (McCarthy and Smith, 2003). In assimilation or harmony deviations: phoneme or syllable is changed to become more similar to another phoneme or syllable in the word. The influence of one phoneme or syllable upon other phonemes or syllables in a word can be from left to right or from right to left. Progressive assimilation occurs when a sound in a word is influenced by a preceding phoneme e.g. 'doggy'→ [doddy]. Regressive assimilation occurs when a phoneme is influenced by a later phoneme e.g. 'doggy'→ [goggy]. Assimilation can be contiguous (influencing sound is adjacent to the changed phoneme) or non-contiguous (influencing phoneme is not adjacent to the changed phoneme).

Assimilation occurs even when the influencing phoneme is omitted in the production (Hodson, 2004). Different types of assimilation appear in the speech of children that can be classified as consonant, voicing and syllable assimilation or harmony. Most of these deviations have been noted in children who are developing speech normally.

I – Consonant Assimilation:

Consonant assimilation can be analysed according to place feature (labial, alveolar, palatal, velar or any place of consonant articulation) or manner feature (nasal, stop, fricative). It may occur in progressive and regressive forms; e.g. labial assimilation occurs when a non-labial sound is changed to a labial in the presence of a labial sound either preceding or following the affected consonant in the adult standard production of the word. An example of progressive labial assimilation is 'boat'→ [bob] and of regressive labial assimilation is 'thumb' → [wʌm].

Regressive contiguous assimilation was found to have the highest frequency in word shapes containing two contiguous consonants e.g. (cvc, cvc). This type is termed local assimilation where strictly adjacent segments become similar (Aboelsaad et al., 2018). Phonetically, local assimilation may be attributed to the minimisation of articulatory effort, i.e. to avoid unnecessary shifts in structure or place of articulation within a sequence of segments (Youssef, 2013).

II – Voicing Assimilation:

Voicing deviations are not always considered assimilation error patterns, but rather are simply categorised as voicing phonological deviations. Two types of voicing assimilation are commonly reported in English children including prevocalic voicing and final consonant devoicing. Prevocalic voicing refers to voicing an unvoiced consonant when it precedes a vowel. What seems to be happening is the voicing of the vowel influences and the voicing feature of the preceding consonant, e.g. 'pig'→ [big] and 'tag' →[dæg]. Postvocalic devoicing is changing a voiced obstruent at the end of a word to a voiceless obstruent. Reportedly; it is the most frequent type of voicing alteration occurring often in conjunction with a slight vowel prolongation, e.g. 'pig' → [pik] and 'bees' → [bis] (Hodson, 2004; Hodson and Paden, 1991). The other two possibilities of voicing errors, such as prevocalic devoicing and postvocalic voicing occur infrequently and are considered unusual patterns. Prevocalic devoicing is the deviation in which a voiced consonant sound that precedes a vowel is changed to a voiceless consonant. Theoretically because of the influence of the silence preceding it.

III – Syllable Assimilation:

Reduplication is a syllable harmony or assimilation deviation in which all or part of a syllable is repeated. Reduplication can occur in complete and partial forms. Examples of complete reduplication are 'water'→ [wɑwɑ]. Examples of partial reduplication include 'doggie' → [dɑdi]. This deviation tends to occur in the speech of young children who have an expressive vocabulary of 50 or fewer words.

3-Feature Contrast or Substitution Error Patterns

These deviations involve replacing one sound by another sound without being influenced by the surrounding phonemes. The substitutions generally are of one class of phonemes replacing another class of phonemes. These deviations affect liquids, stops, fricatives, affricates, nasals and glides and most of them occur in the speech of typically developing children.

I – Stopping:

Stopping has been described with slight variations by phonologists. Khan (1982) described it as substitution of stops for fricatives and affricates. Bankson and Bernthal (1990) described it as stops replacing fricatives, affricates, glides and liquids. Hodson and Paden (1991) defined it as a substitution of a continuant phoneme by a stop, affricate or nasal. This criterion reflects the identification of stops, affricates, nasals as non-continuant.

Stopping is a commonly used process particularly for fricatives, e.g. 'zoo' → [du] (Hodson and Paden, 1991). This error pattern occurs when a fricative is replaced by a stop consonant that shares the same place of articulation (homorganic stop). If there is no homorganic stop, then replacement is by a stop at the nearest place of articulation. Thus, labiodental fricatives (/f/ and /v/) are replaced by labial stops ([p] and [b]), while interdental fricatives (/θ/ and /ð/), alveolar fricatives (/s/ and /z/) and palatal fricatives or affricates (/ʃ/, /ʒ/, /tʃ/ and /dʒ/) are all replaced by alveolar stops ([t] and [d]) (Kirk and Vigeland,2015).

Positional asymmetries have been reported for the stopping of fricatives and affricates such that stopping is more common for word-initial fricatives and affricates than for word-final fricatives and affricates (Smit, 1993). Although many phonologists consider substituting stops for affricates to be stopping, Hodson (2004) indicated that such substitutions should not be classified as stopping because affricates already contain a stop component. Rather, they prefer to describe the replacement of an affricate with a stop as deaffrication. Similarly, the replacement of a fricative or affricate by a glottal stop should not be classified as stopping, given that glottal stop replacement affects a much wider class of consonants than just fricatives and affricates (James, 2001). Some researchers have classified /h/ as a glide along with /j/ and /w/ and argues that /h/ is rarely replaced by a stop in the speech of young children (Smit, 1993). Whatever, stopping can be defined as replacing a continuant phoneme by a non-continuant one.

II – Fronting:

Fronting refers to the replacement of a target phoneme with another phoneme that is articulated anteriorly to the target phoneme (Hodson, 2004). Dyson and Paden (1983) described fronting as replacement of velar or palatal consonant by a phoneme produced farther forward in the mouth than the target.

A-Velar Fronting:

Although some phonologists (e.g. Inkelas and Rose, 2007; McAllister Byun, 2012) have defined velar fronting as

53

occurring when a velar consonant is replaced by a coronal consonant (alveolar and interdentals). Others (e.g. Dyson, 1986; James, 2001) adopted a stricter definition of velar fronting such that velars are replaced by alveolar only, e.g. 'game' → [dem]. Fronting of word-initial velars is much more common than fronting of word-final velars (Smit, 1993; Inkelas and Rose, 2007).

B-Palatal Fronting:

The error pattern of palatal fronting occurs when a palatal phoneme is replaced by an alveolar phoneme, e.g. 'sheep' → [sip] (Kirk and Vigeland, 2015). Palatal fronting should be assessed independently from the fronting of velars, given that velar fronting resolves earlier than palatal fronting in typically developing children (Stoel-Gammon and Dunn, 1985).

III – Affrication (Aff):

Affrication occurs when a stop component is added to a continuant consonant, most commonly a fricative, i.e. a non-affricate becomes an affricate, e.g. 'show' → [tʃo].

IV – Deaffrication:

Deaffrication is the process of replacing an affricate with a non-affricate, i.e. changing an affricate to a continuant or a stop, e.g. 'chair' → [ʃɛr] or [tɛr] (Hodson and Paden, 1991).

V – Palatalisation:

Palatalisation occurs when a sound is produced as a palatal rather than as a non-palatal, e.g. 'soup'→ [ʃup] (Hodson and Paden, 1991). For example, a child's production of [ʃip] for 'sip' could be labelled as backing or palatalisation. Either error pattern would be correct, however, the error pattern of palatalisation provides a more precise description of what the child is doing rather than the broader process of backing (Dodd, 2011).

VI – Depalatalisation:

Depalatalisation is the opposite of palatalisation in that a palatal consonant is replaced by a non-palatal, e.g. 'mash' → [mæs]. As before, more than one phonological error pattern can be used to label an error sometimes this phonological deviation is called "palatal fronting". But, depalatalisation is a more general name as it means the replacement of palatal phonemes by not only alveolar but also labial and labiodental phonemes.

VII – Gliding:

This error pattern of gliding occurs when a glide (/w/ or /j/) replaces a liquid (/r/ or /l/), e.g. 'rain'→ [wen] and 'little'→ [jitl]. For most children, gliding of /l/ resolves earlier than gliding of /r/. Although other consonants (e.g. fricatives) are sometimes replaced by glides, this occurs rarely in the speech of children with typical phonological development as well as those with a phonological disorders (Smit, 1993).

VIII – Vowelisation (Vocalisation):

Vowelisation means production of a vowel for a consonant; usually for a postvocalic liquid, e.g. 'star'→ [stɑʊ] (Miccio and Scarpino, 2009).

IX – Glottal Replacement:

Glottal stop /ʔ/ is not a distinctive phoneme in the English language and thus it serves as a marker for an omitted consonant. This deviation can be classified as a feature contrast or substitution pattern defined as substituting a glottal stop for a consonant usually in the medial or final position e.g. 'fishing' → [fiʔiŋ] and 'bath' → [bɑʔ]. This deviation does not occur frequently in the speech of the typically developing English children. However, it should be noted that /ʔ/is a distinctive phoneme in some other languages and a few English dialects. For instance, the /ʔ/ sound is a unique Arabic phoneme and glottal replacement is very common in Arabic children in any word position (Amayreh and Dyson, 2000; Saleh et al., 2007).

4-Others:

A – Unusual Error Patterns:

Unusual error patterns are error patterns that are unique to a child's phonological system, (table 2) (Khan, 1982). The phonological error pattern of a young child might be unique or rare as it is either not occurring or rarely occurring in the phonologies of other children or of other languages (Leonard and Brown, 1984).

Table 2: Unusual Error Patterns
(Gordon-Brannan and Weiss, 2007)

Process	Definition
Atypical Cluster Reduction	Deletion of the cluster member that is usually retained, e.g. 'train' → [ren].
Initial Consonant Deletion	Deletion of a word initial consonant or cluster, so that the word starts with a vowel, e.g. 'coat' → [ot].
Metathesis	Reversing consonants in a word without changing CV structure of the word, e.g. 'animal' → [æminʊl].
Migration	Movement of a phoneme from one position in the word to another position with changing CV structure of the word, e.g. 'spoon'→ [puns].
Apicalisation	A labial consonant is replaced by a tongue-tip (apical) consonant, e.g. 'bow'→ [dou].
Backing of stops	Replacement of front stops with another stop whose place of articulation is

	posterior to it (typically velars), e.g. 'toe'→ [ko].
Backing of fricatives	Replacement of front fricatives with a fricative made posterior to it, e.g. 'suit'→ [ʃit].
Denasalisation	A nasal is replaced by a homorganic non-nasal sound mostly a stop, e.g. 'man'→ [bæn].
Fricative replacing stops	Substitution of a fricative for a stop, e.g. 'doll'→ [zol].
Stops replacing glides	Substitution of a stop for a glide, e.g. 'wet' → [bet].
Sound preference substitutions	Replacement of groups of consonants by one or two particular consonants, e.g. (/s/,/z/,/ʃ/,/tʃ/,/dʒ/)→[t].
Glottal Replacement	Substituting a glottal stop for a consonant usually in the medial or final position, e.g. 'bath' → [bɑʔ].

❖ **Systematic sound preference** *(Sound preference substitutions):*

Yavas and Hernandorena (1991) stated that systematic sound preference occurs when a group of sounds with the same manner of articulation is represented by one or two sounds in the production of the child. Systematic sound preference is considered one error pattern, although by its very nature it includes various error patterns. Since it involves the loss of several contrasts (because the child utilises one sound for various targets) it implies a severe disorder. There are four hypotheses regarding systematic sound preference:

1. It affects a class of sounds with the same manner of articulation.
2. Fricatives are affected more frequently than any other class of sounds.
3. It is limited to a single position in the word, more commonly word-initial position.
4. When only some members of a class of sounds are affected, voiceless and/ or non-labial sounds are more frequently affected.

B – Articulatory shifts:

Hodson (1980) identified some error patterns which she labelled articulatory shifts in which there are "minimal shifts in place of articulation, while, manner of articulation is the same". These error patterns are often "normal developmental misarticulation" and as Hodson, 1980 indicated, these shifts alone not greatly affect the intelligibility. There are four types of articulatory shifts, first substitution of/f, v, s, z/ for /Ɵ/, e.g. 'mouth' → [mæus]. A second type is frontal lisp which is producing/s/ and sometimes/ ʃ, z, tʃ, dʒ / with protruded tongue i.e. with tongue placement being too far forward. Third type is dentalisation of / t, d, n, l / in which these phonemes are produced with a tongue protrusion. The fourth type of articulatory shift pattern is lateralisation in which air is emitted laterally through the teeth rather than medially. This occurs primarily on the sibilants.

Age of Suppression of Phonological Error Patterns

According to natural phonology, there seems to be a time frame during which normally developing children suppress certain error patterns. This approximate age of suppression is helpful when determining normal versus disordered phonological system and can be used as guidelines when targeting remediation goals. Use of phonological error patterns is typically discontinued by the time the child reaches a certain developmental age. This suppression occurs through a series of steps. Usually at the early stages, such rules are very broad, applying to a whole class of sounds. As the child develops phonological skills, obligatory rules may become optional, being used only part of the time even in the same word (Dyson and Paden 1983). The age of an error pattern suppression was defined by Lowe (1986) as the earliest age at which 90% of a certain age group and all later age groups achieved suppression of the error pattern. The ages by which the child discontinues the use of phonological error patterns has been shown to vary by language (So and Dodd, 1995). Roberts et al. (1990) found that error patterns resolved rapidly between 2½ and 4 years typically developing English children. Owaida (2015) reported that Syrian-Arabic children no longer produce developmental error patterns by the age of 5½ years. Also (Aboelsaad et al., 2018) reported that by the age of 5 years, all phonological error patterns in Egyptian-Arabic children will disappear except postvccalic voicing.

Methods of Assessment of Phonological Error Patterns

Collected speech sample from the examined children can be spontaneous or elicited (table 3). Using tasks that encompass both a naming and imitated task can be important because they allow children to show their linguistic abilities with and without a clinician model and with context through pictures (Hale-Haniff and Siegel, 1981).

Table 3: Methods Used to Collect a Speech Sample
(Bleile, 2004)

Methods	Definition
Spontaneous Speech	Naturally occurring speech
Elicited Speech Naming	Single words typically elicited through naming objects or pictures.

Sentence Completion	Single words typically elicited through the child finishing the clinician's sentence.
Delayed Imitation	Single words typically elicited through placing a short phrase between the clinician's model and the child's response.
Imitation	Single words typically elicited through the child's immediate imitation of the clinician's model.

Before starting the assessment of a child's phonological error patterns, the clinician should decide which measure either single word testing or conversational speech sample is suitable as each measure has advantages and disadvantages. The majority of clinicians always prefer a norm-referenced single-word test (table 4) for assessment (Skahan et al., 2007).

The advantages of single word testing are:

1. It is simple and easy to administer.
2. The clinicians can control word lists to be specially designed to elicit sounds in a variety of word positions and phonetic contexts.
3. The test has definite words so it is helpful to expect and transcribe speech of a highly unintelligible child.
4. It facilitates comparison between children or in one child longitudinally, because data are based on a single measure.

The disadvantage of single-word testing often discussed is that naming may overestimate a child's true abilities and thus fail to reflect his performance in real-life communication (Wolk and Meisler, 1998).

Spontaneous speech samples for assessment of phonological error patterns has some advantages:

1. Reflect the child's performance in the most real-life natural communication. This method is strengthened by the availability of phonetic contexts which are thought to be important in phonological assessment (Wolk and Meisler, 1998).
2. Spontaneous speech sample is comprehensive. Some single word tests do not include many polysyllabic words and the examiner need to look beyond those tests for a comprehensive sample (Baker et al., 2011).
3. Children may enjoy the assessment process of spontaneous speech sample as it is a self-made measure and may incorporate current events and popular characters.
4. Other advantages like it is a cheap and available method. So, spontaneous speech sampling may be used when single word tests are inappropriate or not available (Joffe and Pring, 2008).

However, in spite of these important advantages, spontaneous speech sampling has some disadvantages:

1. Sometimes, children may be unwilling to cooperate or may be too shy to engage in spontaneous conversation, or may have behavioural complications which make it impossible.
2. Moreover, speech output from a highly unintelligible child may be difficult to transcribe or it may be difficult for the clinician to determine the target word.
3. Children may intentionally avoid certain sounds with which they know they have difficulty or avoid certain phonetic contexts.
4. The sample will be different both between and within children. This can cause problems in research and make it more difficult for a clinician to evaluate a child's performance systematically over time, thus limiting prognostic and treatment outcome evaluations (Wolk and Meisler, 1998).

Age-Appropriate Speech Sampling Tasks (Stein-Rubin and Fabus, 2011)

According to Kamhi (2005), a useful spontaneous speech sample should contain a minimum of 100 different words. There are many tasks that can be used for spontaneous speech sampling:

For younger children: Wordless picture books; telling back a story; play activities; counting 1 to 10, reciting ABCs; describing a favourite birthday party, a special fun time or a favourite vacation and describing a contextual picture with lots of action.

For older children: Conversing about a TV show, school subject, magazine article, sports or hobby; discussing favourite parts of school or favourite activities and describing how to play a certain sport or make a particular craft item.

Masterson et al. (2005) looked at 20 children's spontaneous speech samples and compared them to their single-word samples. All participants were administered the Computerised Articulation and Phonology Evaluation System (Masterson and Bernhardt, 2001) that contained single words partially adapted to match the phonological system of each individual participant. Results revealed no major differences of the participants' speech production abilities between that of the spontaneous speech sample and the single-word samples. Their findings suggest that using single-word samples can be an effective and faster way to evaluate a child's speech sound system than collecting and analysing a larger speech sample.

Selection Criteria for Target Words Used in the Assessment of Phonological Error Patterns

Some phonologists may use articulation tests for assessment of both articulation and phonological error patterns. However, most articulation tests describe the sound system in terms of substitutions and distortions in word–initial, medial and final positions (i.e. assesses the production of consonants and vowels). On the other hand, phonological tests target sound classes, sound sequences and different syllable structure with sufficient opportunities (Lowe, 1986). An articulation test can be a phonological test depending on the manner in which the researcher analyses the results. For example, if he looks at speech sound classes and attempts to find out the phonological error patterns that apply to them, then the test will be phonological (Owaida, 2015).

Hodson (2006) stated some criteria for choosing target words; the words should be familiar to children; can be elicited by objects or pictures; the words should provide at least 10 opportunities for occurrences of each of the target phonological error patterns; Each word may provide opportunities for assessing more than one phonological error patterns: All consonants and vowels should be included; The target words should contain monosyllabic, disyllabic and multisyllabic words.

It is very important for clinicians designing single-word naming test to choose phonetically simple words to assess phonological error patterns. However, this could be criticised, as it does not provide a complete picture of a child's phonological system as error patterns in the speech of older children are more likely to show up in words consisting of three or more syllables than in shorter words (James et al., 2008). So that, single-word tests should include polysyllabic words to be more comprehensive (Baker et al., 2011).

When assessing the production of word-final consonants, it is important that consonants with different manners and places of articulation be included. However, neither the lateral liquid nor the rhotic liquid should be included as opportunities for the error pattern of final consonant deletion (FCD) because postvocalic /l/ is often vocalised in adult speech and so does not provide a valid opportunity for assessing the production of word-final consonants (Schneider et al., 2004).

Any valid measure of the error pattern of cluster reduction should sample both word-initial clusters and word-final clusters because only by comparing the production of words such as blocks and box, we can determine whether the child's inability to say the final cluster in these words is due to a phonological impairment or to an impairment in grammatical morphology (Kirk and Vigeland, 2015).

In addition to expanding the number of opportunities for some error patterns, test developers should consider eliminating error patterns that are unlikely to be helpful in determining appropriate intervention targets. For example, the error pattern of deaffrication occurs so rarely for the voiced affricate /ʤ/, so, the inclusion of /ʤ/ as an opportunity for deaffrication may lead to underestimating the percentage of occurrence of this error pattern (Smit, 1993). For this reason, Kirk and Vigeland (2015) recommended including only examples where the voiceless affricate /ʧ/ is replaced with [ʃ] as valid opportunities for deaffrication.

Given the positional asymmetries for stopping of fricatives and affricates, it is important that sufficient opportunities are provided for evaluating these phonemes in word-initial position. Also, the fact that word-initial velars are fronted more commonly than word-final velars, it should be taken into consideration when evaluating the number of opportunities for this error pattern to occur in a child's speech. Given this asymmetry, it is important that a test contains sufficient opportunities for evaluating word-initial velars (Kirk and Vigeland, 2015).

Smit (1993) reported that fronting of palatals occurs frequently in both the word-initial position and the word-final position, suggesting that opportunities for testing this error pattern are likely to be equally represented in either position. Although consonants other than liquids are sometimes replaced by glides, this occurs very infrequently in the speech of children with typical phonological development as well as those with a phonological disorder (Smit, 1993). Therefore, these consonants other than liquids do not provide reasonable opportunities for this error pattern to occur (Kirk and Vigeland, 2015).

An additional consideration is that some error patterns remove the opportunity for another error pattern to occur. For example, a child who reduces all consonant clusters to a singleton consonant is likely to remove opportunities for gliding of liquids in words such as blue and crab. So, the total number of opportunities for gliding will need to be adjusted, or the percentage of occurrence for the error pattern of gliding will be misrepresented (Kirk and Vigeland, 2015).

Before we can determine whether single-word tests provide a sufficient number of opportunities to establish the various phonological error patterns in a child's speech, it is necessary to come up with a set of core phonological error patterns and provide recommendations on the best way to evaluate each of them (Kirk and Vigeland, 2015).

It is the responsibility of clinicians working with children from culturally and linguistically diverse populations to familiarise themselves with the phonological features of the specific dialect spoken by their clients to avoid misdiagnosing phonological differences as a speech sound disorder (ASHA, 2004).

Table 4: Summary of Commonly Administered Tests of Phonology

Authors of Test	Hodson (2004)	Dawson and Tattersall (2001)	Khan and Lewis (2015)	Bankson and Bernthal (1990)	Secord and Donohue (2014)	Dodd, Hua, Crosbie, Holm and Ozanne (2009)	Lowe (1986)	Abou-Elsaad, Afsah and Rabea (2018)
Name of the test	Hodson Assessment of Phonological Patterns, 3rd ed. (HAAP-3)	Structured Photographic Articulation Test II featuring Dudsberry the Golden Retriever (SPAT-D II)	Khan-Lewis Phonological Analysis, Third Edition (KLPA-3)	Bankson-Bernthal Test of Phonology (BBTOP)	Clinical Assessment of Articulation and Phonology, 2nd ed. (CAAP-2)	Diagnostic Evaluation of Articulation and Phonology (DEAP)	Assessment Link b/w phonology & articulation (ALPHA)	Mansoura Arabic Test for Phonological error patterns (MATPP)
Stimuli	Objects and Pictures	Pictures	from the Goldman Fristoe Test of articulation	Pictures	Pictures	Pictures	Pictures	Pictures
Elicitation method	Object or Picture naming	Picture naming	Picture naming	Picture naming	Picture naming	Picture naming	Sentence imitation	Picture naming
Sample size transcription	50 word	48 words	53 words	80 words	84 words	50 words	50 words	50 words
NO. of phonological error patterns	25 Major Phonological error patterns	7 Phonological error patterns	10 Phonological error patterns	10 Phonological error patterns	10 Phonological error patterns	10 Phonological error patterns	15 Phonological error patterns	8 Phonological error patterns
Target population	Normal and phonological disordered children	Normal and phonological disordered children	Normal and phonological disordered children	Normal and phonological disordered children	Normal and phonological disordered children	Normal and phonological disordered children	Normal and phonological disordered children	Normal and phonological disordered children
Total Time	15-20 min	15 min	10-30 min	15 to 20 min	15–20 min	10-15 min	10-15 min	15-20-min
Age range (yrs months)	3;0 to 7;11	3;0 to 9;11	2;0 to 21;11	3;0 to 9;11	2;6 to 11;11	3;0 to 8;11	3;0 to 8;11	2;0 to 5;0
Area Assessed	Phonological error patterns	Articulation; Phonological error patterns	Phonological error patterns	Articulation; Phonological error patterns	Articulation; Phonological error patterns	Articulation; Phonological error patterns	Articulation; Phonological error patterns	Phonological error patterns

Phonetic Transcription

Phonetic transcription is the use of phonetic symbols to represent speech sounds. Ideally, each sound in a spoken utterance is represented by a written phonetic symbol. The transcription system will in general reflect the phonetic analysis imposed by the transcriber on the material. In particular, the choice of symbol set will tend to reflect decisions about segmentation of the language data and its phonological treatment (Wells, 2006).

The International Phonetic Alphabet (IPA) is used to describe the different sounds in child speech. The IPA is a group of speech sound symbols selected to represent the broadest consensus of articulatory characteristics across the world's languages (Stein-Rubin and Fabus, 2011). There are generally two types of transcription that could be used to transcribe a child's speech: broad and narrow phonetic transcription (Bauman-Waengler, 2008). To transcribe the child's speech, the sounds are placed within brackets (broad phonetic transcription); however, special symbols or diacritic may be used to further explain the child's speech (narrow phonetic transcription). Diacritics are used to mark the allophonic variations of a sound (Heselwood and Howard, 2008).

Transcription of live speech has advantage of being listened to in its natural state, but it is unreliable because it is impossible to write the symbols and diacritics down at the speed at which the speaker produces sounds, asking a speaker to repeat a lexical item is often undertaken with intra-speaker variability and it is harder to ignore the linguistic aspects of the speech and to concentrate only on the sounds. The problems of subjectivity and unreliability can be solved by controlling the conditions under which a transcription is made but still constrained by the biological and cognitive limitations of our perceptual abilities (Heselwood and Howard, 2009).

The first necessity is to record the speech sample on a good-quality recording system so that the transcription can be made from listening to a recording. A video recording is better than audio recording as silent articulation (mouthing) is an important phonetic behaviour in impaired speech which will not be evident on audio recordings. Once a recording is made, the next consideration is how best to listen (Heselwood and Howard, 2009). Ladefoged (2003) recommended listening through headphones "as this is better than free-field listening" and using a reverse-play function "to focus more easily on phonetic structure of the speaker's output".

Analysis Methods

Independent and relational analyses are procedures used in the clinical assessment of children's single word and/or spontaneous speech samples (Cohen and Anderson, 2011). Independent analysis explores and identifies the consonants and vowels, syllable-word shapes and syllable-stress patterns that a child can produce regardless of accuracy and its relationship to the adult target (Baker and Bernhardt, 2004). Relational analysis compares the child's productions with the adult target and involves determining the pattern of errors and consistency of the productions relative to the target (Williams, 2003).

According to a survey conducted by Skahan et al. (2007), phonological error pattern analysis is the most commonly used speech sound analysis procedure administered by speech language pathologists and phoniatricians. This type of analysis is recommended for children with multiple speech errors as part of a comprehensive assessment of SSD (Bernthal et al., 2013). Bou (2008) developed the ABC method for analysing phonological patterns. It is drawn from the main areas of speech composition; syllables, intra-syllabic structures and sound structure.

The *ABC* Method is based on that a good analysis will lead to a more target specific treatment. It can be both applied to the phonological evaluation procedure as well as during the course of treatment to evaluate treatment efficacy. After taking and transcribing the speech sample, the clinician applies steps A, B and C to the analysis of patterns. Each step considers each level of the word structure and is based on the same areas as phonological awareness (Gillon, 2004).

In *step A*: The clinician will look at the quantity of syllables produced by the child and will compare this quantity with the number of syllables within the target word. In this step the clinician is looking for syllable structure error patterns that affect the number of syllables in a word (e.g. syllable deletion).

In *step B:* Clinicians will be looking for patterns that affect mostly syllable onset and coda (e.g. initial consonant deletion, final consonant deletion, cluster reduction).

In *step C:* The clinician will analyse changes in segment features. In this step substitution error patterns are specified as they relate to changes in manner, place or voicing (e.g. fronting, stopping and backing).

The analysis of a word based on its syllable structure yield more accurate and clinically valid results than the analysis of a word by its beginning-initial, middle-medial and end-final sound position (Bauman-Waengler, 2008).

Chapter Summary

Phonological error patterns are a systematic change in sound class or cluster or syllable. Concerning its tendency to affect certain groups of phonological elements, it should occur twice at least to classify it as phonological error patterns. In this chapter, phonological error patterns are classified into four main types: syllable structure error patterns; assimilation error patterns; substitution error patterns and others including unusual error patterns and developmental articulatory shifts. How to assess phonological error patterns either by spontaneous sample speech or by single word test is discussed also besides advantages and disadvantages of each measure. Selection criteria of target words for simple word testing are also described, in addition to phonetic transcription and methods of pattern analysis in this chapter.

References

Abell, A. (2006). Diagnostic evaluation of articulation and phonology (DEAP).

Abou-Elsaad, T., Afsah, O., & Rabea, M. (2018). Identification of Phonological Processes in Arabic–Speaking Egyptian Children by Single-word Test. Journal of communication disorders.

Amayreh, M and Dyson, A (2000): Phonological errors and sound changes in Arabic-speaking children. Clinical linguistics and phonetics, 14, 79-109.

American Speech-Language-Hearing Association. (2004): preferred practice patterns for the profession of speech-language pathology: #15, Speech sound assessment. Rockville, MD: ASHA. Retrieved from http://www. Asha.org/policy.

Baker, E., and McLeod, S. (2011). Evidence-based practice for children with speech sound disorders: Part 1 narrative review. Language, Speech, and Hearing Services in Schools, 42(2), 102-139.

Bankson, N. W., and Bernthal, J. E. (1990). Bankson-Bernthal test of phonology. Applied Symbolix.

Baunm-Waengler, J. (2004). Articulatory and Phonological Impairments: A clinical focus (2nd Ed.). Boston: Allyn and Bacon.

Bauman-Waengler, J. (2008): Articulatory and phonological impairments: A clinical focus (3rd Ed.). Boston: Allyn and Bacon.

Bernthal, J. E., Bankson, N. W., and Flipsen, P. (2013): Articulation and phonological disorders: Speech sound disorders in children (7th ed.). Upper Saddle River, NJ: Pearson.

Bleile, K. M. (2004). Manual of Articulation and Phonological Disorders: Infancy through adulthood (2nd ed.). Clinical Competence Series. Clifton Park, NY: Delmar/Cengage Learning.

Bloch, T. (2011). Simplification Strategies in the Acquisition of Consonant Clusters in Hebrew (Doctoral dissertation, Tel-Aviv University).

Bosch Galceran, L. (2004). Phonological Assessment of Children's Speech. Barcelona: Masson.

Bou, L. (2008): Spanish phonological patterns identification and analysis. Poster Number 266, Session 1862 presented at the meeting of the American Speech-Language and Hearing Association (ASHA) Annual Convention Chicago, 2008.

Carter, A. K., and Gerken, L. (2003). Similarities in weak syllable omissions between children with specific language impairment and normally developing language: a preliminary report. Journal of Communication Disorders, 36(2), 165-179.

Cohen, W., and Anderson, C. (2011): Identification of phonological processes in preschool children's single-word productions. International Journal of Language & Communication Disorders, 46(4), 481-488.

Dawson J. and Tattersall B. (2001): Structured Photographic Articulation Test (2nd Ed.) JP. Creative. Speech and Language Materials. Featuring Dudsberry. DeKalb, IL: Janelle Publishing.

Dodd, B., 2011: Differentiating speech delay from disorder. Does it matter? Topics in Language Disorders, 31(2), 96–111.

Dodd, B., Holm, A., Hua, Z. and Crosbie, S. (2003). Phonological development: a normative study of British English-speaking children. Clinical Linguistics & Phonetics, 17(8), 617-643.

Dodd, B., Holm, A., Hua, Z. and Crosbie, S. (2003): Phonological development: a normative study of

British English-speaking children. Clinical Linguistics & Phonetics, 17(8), 617-643.

Dodd, B., Hua, Z., Crosbie, S., Holm, A., & Ozanne, A. (2009). Diagnostic Evaluation of Articulation and Phonology—US Edition (DEAP). San Antonio, TX: Pearson.

Dyson, A. T. (1986): Development of velar consonants among normal two-year-olds. Journal of Speech and Hearing Research, 29, 493–498.

Dyson, A. T., and Paden, E. P. (1983): Some phonological acquisition strategies used by two-year-olds. Communication Disorders Quarterly, 7(1), 6-18.

Gillon, G. T. (2004). Phonological Awareness: From Research to Practice (New York, NY: Guilford).

Gammon, C., and Dunn, C. (1985): Normal and disordered phonology in children. Pro Ed.

Gordon-Brannan, M. E., & Weiss, C. E. (2007). Clinical management of articulatory and phonologic disorders. Lippincott Williams & Wilkins.

Hale-Haniff, M., and Siegel, G. M. (1981): The effect of context on verbal elicited imitation. Journal of Speech and Hearing Disorders, 46(1), 27-30.

Heselwood, B. and Howard, S., (2008): Clinical phonetic transcription. In M.J. Ball, M. Perkins, N. Mueller, and S. Howard (eds), The handbook of clinical linguistics (Oxford: Blackwell), pp.381-399.

Heselwood, B., and Howard, S. (2009): 23 Clinical Phonetic Transcription. The handbook of clinical linguistics, 56, 381.

Hodson, B. W. (1980): The Assessment of Phonological Processes. Danville, IL: Interstate.

Hodson, B.W. (2004). Hodson Assessment of Phonological Patterns. East Moline, IL: Linguisystems.

Hodson B. W. (2006): Identifying phonological patterns and projecting remediation cycles: Expediting intelligibility gains of a 7-year-old Australian child.

Advances in Speech–Language Pathology; 8(3): 257–264.

Hodson, B. W., and Paden, E. P. (1981): Phonological processes which characterize unintelligible and intelligible speech in early childhood. Journal of Speech and Hearing Disorders, 46, 369–373.

Hodson, B. W., and Paden, E. P. (1991). A phonological approach to remediation: Targeting intelligible speech. Austin, TX: Pro Ed.

Ingram, D. (1989). First language acquisition: Method, description and explanation. Cambridge University Press.

Inkelas, S., and Rose, Y. (2007): Positional neutralization: A case study from child language. Language, 707-736.

James, D. G. (2001): Use of phonological processes in Australian children ages 2 to 7; 11 years. Advances in Speech Language Pathology, 3(2), 109-127.

James, D. G. H., van Doorn, J., and McLeod, S. (2008): The contribution of polysyllabic words in clinical decision making about children's speech. Clinical Linguistics & Phonetics, 22, 345–353.

Joffe, V., and Pring, T. (2008). Children with phonological problems: A survey of clinical practice. International Journal of Language and Communication Disorders, 43, 154–164.

Kamhi, A. G. (2005): In Alan G. Kamhi & Karen E. Pollack (Eds.), Phonological disorders in children: Clinical decision making in assessment and intervention. Baltimore, MD: Brookes Publishing.

Khan, L. (1982). A review of 16 major phonological processes. Language, Speech, & Hearing in Schools, 13, 77–85.

Khan, L., and Lewis, N. (2015): Khan-Lewis phonological analysis (3rd Edition). Pearson Assessment UK.

Kirk, C., and Vigeland, L. (2015). Content coverage of single-word tests used to assess common phonological error patterns. Language, speech, and hearing services in schools, 46(1), 14-29.

Ladefoged, P. (2003). Phonetic data analysis: An introduction to fieldwork and instrumental techniques (pp. 104-137). Malden, MA: Blackwell.

Leonard, L. B., and Brown, B. L. (1984). Nature and Boundaries of Phonologic Categories: A Case Study of an Unusual Phonologic Pattern in a Language-Impaired Child. Journal of Speech and Hearing Disorders, 49(4), 419-428.

Lowe, R. J. (1986): ALPHA: Assessment Link between Phonology and Articulation. LinguiSystems, Incorporated.

Lowe, R. J. (1996): Assessment link between phonology and articulation: ALPHA (rev. ed.). Mifflinville, PA: Speech and Language Resources.

Masterson, J. J., & Bernhardt, B. H., (2001). Computerized articulation and phonology evaluation system (CAPES). San Antonio, TX: The Psychological Corporation.

Masterson, J. J., Bernhardt, B. H., and Hofheinz, M. K. (2005): A comparison of single words and conversational speech in phonological evaluation. American Journal of Speech-Language Pathology, 14(3), 229-241

McAllister Byun, T. (2012): Positional velar fronting: An updated articulatory account. Journal of Child Language, 39, 1043–1076.

McCarthy, J. J. and Smith, N. (2003). Phonological processes: Assimilation. In W. Frawley, ed. Oxford International Encyclopaedia of Linguistics. 2nd ed. Oxford: Oxford University Press, 320–3.

McLeod, S., Doorn, J. V., and Reed, V. A. (1997). Realizations of consonant clusters by children with phonological impairment. Clinical Linguistics & Phonetics, 11(2), 85-113.

McReynolds, L. V., and Elbert, M. (1981). Criteria for phonological process analysis. Journal of Speech and Hearing Disorders, 46, 197–204.

Miccio, A. W., and Scarpino, S. E. (2009). 25 Phonological Analysis, Phonological Processes. The handbook of clinical linguistics, 56, 412.

Morsi, R. (2001): Phonological acquisition of normal Egyptian children from the age of two and half to five years. 15th ICPhS Conference, Barcelona.

Owaida, H. (2015): Speech sound acquisition and phonological error patterns in child speakers of Syrian Arabic: a normative study (Doctoral dissertation, City University London).

Prater, R. J., and Swift, R. W. (1982). Phonological process development with MLU-referenced guidelines. Journal of communication disorders, 15(5), 395-410.

Roberts, J. E., Burchinal, M., and Footo, M. M. (1990). Phonological process decline from 212 to 8 years. Journal of Communication Disorders, 23(3), 205-217.

Saleh, M., Shoeib, R., Hegazi, M., & Ali, P. (2007). Early phonological development in Arabic Egyptian children: 12–30 months. Folia Phoniatrica et Logopaedica, 59(5), 234-240.

Schneider, E. W., Burridge, K., Kortman, B., Mesthrie, R., and Upton, C. (Eds.). (2004). A handbook of varieties of English. Vol. 1: Phonology. Berlin, Germany: Mouton de Gruyter.

Secord, W., and Donohue, J. S. (2014): CAAP-2: Clinical Assessment of Articulation and Phonology-2. Super Duper Publications.

Skahan, S. M., Watson, M., and Lof, G. L. (2007). Speech-language pathologists' assessment practices for children with suspected speech sound disorders: Results of a national survey. American Journal of Speech-Language Pathology, 16(3), 246-259.

Smit, A. B. (1993). Phonologic Error Distributions in the Iowa-Nebraska Articulation Norms Project Consonant Singletons. Journal of Speech,

Language, and Hearing Research, 36(3), 533-547.

So, L. K., and Dodd, B. J. (1995): The acquisition of phonology by Cantonese-speaking children. Journal of child language, 22(03), 473-495.

Stein-Rubin, C., and Fabus, R. (2011). Assessment of articulation and phonological disorders: A Guide to Clinical Assessment and Professional Report Writing in Speech-Language Pathology. Nelson Education.

Stoel-Gammon, C., and Dunn, C. (1985): Normal and disordered phonology in children. Pro Ed.

Wells, J. C. (2006): Phonetic transcription and analysis. Encyclopedia of Language and Linguistics. Amsterdam: Elsevier, 386-396.

Williams, A. L. (2003): Speech disorders resource guide for preschool children. Clifton Park, Y: Delmar Learning.

Wolk, L., and Meisler, A. W. (1993). Phonological assessment: A systematic comparison of conversation and picture naming. Journal of Communication Disorders, 31(4), 291-313.

Yavas, M., and Lamprecht, R. (1988): Processes and intelligibility in disordered phonology. Clinical linguistics & phonetics, 2(4), 329-345.

Youssef, I. (2013). Place assimilation in Arabic: Contrasts, features, and constraints. (Unpublished PhD thesis), University of Tromsø–Tromsø, Norway.

Chapter 4:
Speech Sound Disorders

Chapter Outlines

o Definition.
o Prevalence.
o Speech-processing chain and its breakdowns.
o Phonological characteristics of speech sound disorders.
o Aetiology of speech sound disorders.
o Diagnostic criteria of speech sound disorders.
o Subtypes of speech sound disorders.
o Assessment of speech sound disorders.
o Prognosis of speech sound disorders.

Definition

Speech sound disorders (SSD) is a broad term referring to any combination of difficulties with perception, phonological representation and/or motor production affecting speech intelligibility. SSD can impact the form or the function of speech sounds within a language. Disorders that impact the form of speech sounds are named "articulation disorders" and are associated with structural or motor-based difficulties. Disorders that impact the function of speech sounds (phonemes) are named "phonological disorders", they result from impairments in the phonological representation of speech sounds and speech segments (including phonotactic rules that govern syllable shape, structure and prosody) (American Speech-Language and Hearing Association (ASHA), 2014).

Children with SSD form a heterogeneous group of disorders which differ in severity, underlying aetiology, speech error characteristics, involvement of other aspects of the language and response to treatment (Dodd 2011).

Prevalence

Prevalence data on SSD are problematic because definitions of the disorder are not consistent and numerous studies depends on teacher, parent and/or speech-language pathologist (SLP) reports. Most of the prevalence research that has been published has come from the United Kingdom, Australia and Canada, thus, it may be difficult to decide the extent to which those data can be generalised (ASHA, 2014). At four years of age, the prevalence of SSD in an Australian study was 3.4%, comorbidity with SSD was 40.8% for language disorder and 20.8% for poor pre-literacy skills and was common and more likely to be present in males than females (Eadie et al., 2015).

Speech-Processing Chain and its Breakdowns

Dodd (2013) identified five levels of breakdowns in the speech-processing chain of speech sound disorders (figure 4)

1. **Auditory input:** Including hearing impairment, impaired discrimination between speech sounds or language-learning unstimulating environment.
2. **Phonological:** An impairment of attention, reasoning or memory, or low motivation leading to a linguistic disorder in abstracting the phonological constraints of speech production.
3. **Systematic phonetic:** A breakdown between the phonological system and the articulatory system where the phonetic specifications for speech-sound production are inaccurate (i.e. the blueprint or template for production of a particular sounds would result in distorted articulation, such as a lisp).

4. **Articulatory planning:** An impaired ability to formulate sequences of speech sounds that make up an utterance (i.e. childhood apraxia of speech).
5. **Motor execution:** An impairment of motor execution due to peripheral neurological dysfunction (i.e. dysarthria).

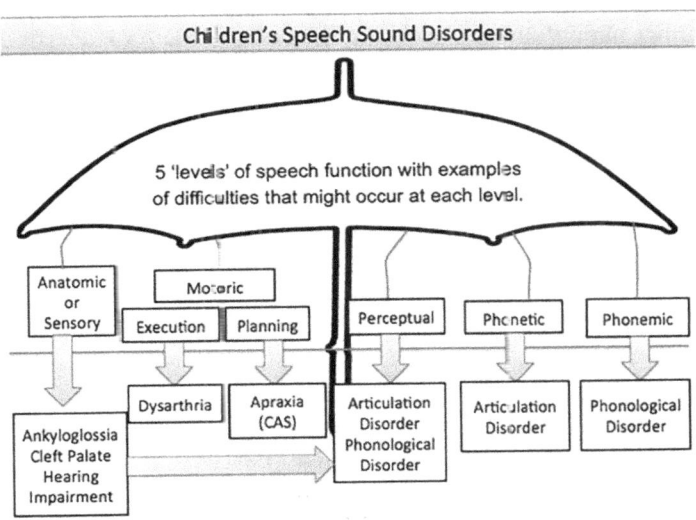

Figure 4: Simple Classification System for 'Underlying Levels' of Difficulty in Speech Sound Disorders
(Bowen, 2015)

Phonological Characteristics of Speech Sound Disorders

From a phonological view, Grunwell (1997) described the characteristics of SSD in terms of system, structure and stability. Specifically, the child's phonological system is smaller than the adult system in which there is an absence of adult phoneme contrasts. This absence results in phoneme collapse, in which the child produces one sound for several different adult sounds. For example, the child produces [t] for

/t/, /k/, /tʃ/, /s/ and /ʃ/, which results in homonymous pronunciations of [tip] for 'tip', 'kip', 'chip', 'sip' and 'ship'. These phoneme collapses are considered as compensatory strategies that the child has developed in order to accommodate his limited or smaller phonological system relative to the larger adult phonological system. In the previous example, the child collapsed voiceless obstruents /t/, /k/, /tʃ/, /s/ and /ʃ/, to a voiceless obstruent [t] that was available in his phonological system (Williams, 2000). As such, there is a relationship between the phonetic properties of the collapsed adult targets and the child's errored substitution and this goes with the generative phonological theory, as applied to children with phonological disorders, argued against assuming that children have adult-like URs, however, according to natural phonology theory assumption, the underlying representation (UR) is to be correct even when production is incorrect. (Dinnsen and Charles-Luce, 1984). With regard to structure, Grunwell (1997) described the child's phonotactic patterns as being more simplistic relative to the structure of the adult phonological system. For example, children with SSD frequently simplify the more complex adult structure of consonant clusters to a singleton. In terms of stability, Grunwell (1997) stated that there is a tendency for some variability in the child's realisations of the adult target. For example, the child might sometimes produce target /k/ as [t] or [g]. This variability might be based on position in the word or syllable in which the target occurs, or it could be influenced by the vowel environment.

Genetic Theory

In medicine, any disease or disorder has a genetic base which interact with certain environmental factors leading to the expression of the disorder. Thus, early screening of the affected genes and environmental modification will prevent expression of the disorder, delay its onset and minimise its severity. Nowadays, Research supports a genetic component to SSD and that holds promise for more understanding of the aetiology. Identifying underlying genetic factors for SSD is very important. Firstly, identification of genetic factors underlying SSD may result in improved diagnosis and early identification of those at risk, allowing for environmental intervention at a young age. Secondly, identifying these factors may lead to the discovery of key genetic pathways (i.e. functional studies of the proteins coded for by specific genes and the resulting metabolic, structural, signalling, transcription regulation, or other cellular pathways), thus bridging the gap between genetics and the neurobiological bases of these disorders. Thirdly, examining and identifying common genetic factors associated with SSD, language impairment (LI) and reading disorders (RD) may assist in the development of meaningful diagnostic categories based on shared underlying deficits, such as impaired phonological representations. Finally, genetic studies of speech and language disorders may provide insight into the evolution of the human capacity for speech and language (Lewis et al., 2006).

Causes of Articulation Disorders

Any breakdowns in the normal prerequisites of articulation development will lead to an articulation disorder. Aetiology of articulation disorders may be organic or functional. Organic causes may result from insult in the structure of the vocal tract or the neurological pathway of speech.

The following are examples of known disorders leading to articulation disorder (ASHA, 2014)

- Structurally based disorders e.g. cleft palate and other craniofacial anomalies.
- Motor-based disorders (apraxia and dysarthria).
- Sensory-based conditions (e.g. hearing impairment).

Functional articulation disorder is diagnosed when there is no apparent cause of the articulation disorder (i.e. structure and innervation of the vocal tract is intact). Any articulation errors persisting beyond age 8 are generally considered residual. Residual errors persist when a motor pattern has been created for a sound or when a structural problem modifies the target place or manner of production (ASHA, 2012).

Causes of Phonological Disorders

Phonological disorder is thought to be caused by an impaired organisation of the phonological system. Any breakdowns in the normal prerequisites of phonemic development will lead to a phonological disorder or both articulation and phonological disorders as the following:

- Sensory-based conditions (e.g. hearing impairment).
- Lack of environmental stimulation for learning.
- Intellectual disabilities.
- Attention disorders.

Diagnostic Criteria of Speech Sound Disorders

- A phonological disorder is characterised by the occurrence of one or more of the following: chronological mismatch of normal error patterns; unusual error patterns; variable use of error patterns; systematic sound preference (Grunwell 1985).
- Edwards and Shriberg (1983) classified a child as having a phonological disorder if he fulfilled either of the following criteria as assessed by a spontaneous speech sample:
1. Exhibited at least two age-inappropriate phonological error patterns and affected at least 25% of all examined words, or
2. Exhibited one or more unusual phonological error patterns and affected at least 25% of all examined words.

- Freiberg and Wicklund (2003) described the identification of a child having SSD by meeting the following criteria:
1. The child's conversational intelligibility is significantly affected and the child displays at least one of the following:
   o The child performs on a norm-referenced test of articulation or phonology at least 1.75 standard deviations below the mean for his chronological age, or
   o Demonstrates consistent articulation errors beyond the time when 90 percent of typically developing children have acquired the sound.
2. One or more of the child's phonological error patterns are occurring at least 40% of all examined words or the child scores in the moderate to profound range of phonological error patterns severity rating in single word testing and the child's conversational intelligibility is significantly affected.

Subtypes of Speech Sound Disorders:

Dodd (2014) classified SSD into five subgroups depended on speech characteristics, underlying subgroup-specific processing deficits and response to therapy (figure 5):

1. *Articulation disorder:* Substitutions or distortions of the same sounds in isolation and in all phonetic contexts during imitation, elicitation and spontaneous speech samples (e.g. lateral lisp) This phonetic disorder affects around 12% of all children with functional SSD and is most successfully treated by traditional articulation therapy.
2. *Phonological delay:* Presence of phonological patterns that are typical of younger children as determined by normative data where fewer than 10% of children in a 6-month age band produced the error in 5 different words on a standard test of 50 words. This phonemic disorder affects around 55% of all

children with functional SSD. Intervention studies indicate that both whole language and phonological contrast intervention are successful approaches to therapy.

3. *Consistent atypical phonological disorder:* Consistent use of one or more unusual error patterns as determined by normative data where fewer than 10% of children, in any age interval, produced the error pattern in five different words on a standard test of 50 words. A child may also display some normal error patterns that are delayed or age-appropriate. This phonemic disorder affects around 20% of all children with functional SSD. Phonological contrast therapy is the only therapeutic approach that has been shown to resolve this SSD.

4. *Inconsistent phonological disorder:* Multiple phonemic error forms for the same lexical item while having no oromotor difficulties, determined by the production of 25 words in three separate trials, with a criterion of 40% for diagnosis of inconsistency (based on normative data of <10% inconsistency for typically developing children and <30% for children with delay or consistent phonological disorder). Children perform better in imitation than spontaneous production. This phonological disorder affects about 10% of children with functional SSD. Core vocabulary therapy that focuses on whole words usually generalises to non-targeted words, establishing consistency and improving accuracy, although follow-up phonological contrast intervention may be indicated once speech is consistent.

5. *Childhood Apraxia of Speech (CAS):* Speech characterised by inconsistency, oromotor signs (e.g. groping, difficulty sequencing articulatory movements), slow speech rate, disturbed prosody, short utterance length, poorer performance in imitation than spontaneous production. It may

involve multiple deficits affecting phonological and phonetic planning as well as motor programme execution

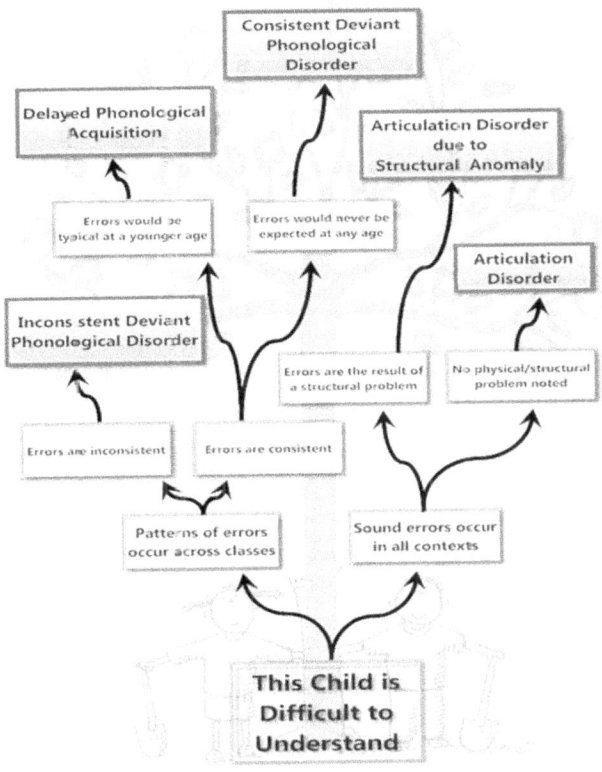

Figure 5: Speech Sound Disorder Tree
(Source: Bilinguistics.Com, 2016)

Assessment of Speech Sound Disorders

• *Purposes of Assessment:*

The reasons behind why clinicians assess children's speech is an essential precursor to considering which measures are used and how they are selected (Leitão, 2011).

The clinician may assess children's speech production for a number of purposes including screening, diagnosing, selecting intervention targets, monitoring progress and determining when to discharge. However, screening and diagnosing are the two main reasons (Bankson et al., 2009).

- ### *Screening:*

Screening aims to differentiate between normal children and children with SSD who require more comprehensive assessment. It is conducted whenever SSD is suspected or as part of a comprehensive speech and language evaluation for a child with communication disorders (ASHA, 2014).

- ### *Approach to Diagnosis of Speech Sound Disorders:*

Diagnostic assessment comprises more comprehensive sampling of children's speech and its results indicate the presence and severity of speech impairment. They also provide information about skills to be targeted and possible strategies to be planned in therapy (Bankson et al., 2009).

ASHA (2014) described the comprehensive assessment for SSD (figure 7) including case history, vocal tract examination, hearing screening, speech sound assessment, spoken-language testing, phonological processing and literacy assessment.

1. Case History:

The case history includes collecting information about family's concerns about the child's speech, history of middle ear infections, languages used in the home, primary language spoken by the child, history of speech, language and/or literacy difficulties in the family, family's perception of intelligibility and teacher's perception of the child's intelligibility and child's performance in comparison to his peers in the classroom.

2. Vocal Tract Examination:

The vocal tract examination evaluates the structure and function of the speech mechanism to assess whether the system is appropriate for speech production. This examination includes assessment of occlusion and specific tooth deviations, hard and soft palate (clefts, fistulas, bifid uvula), function (strength and range of motion) of the lips, jaw, tongue and velum, placement of the tongue at rest and during speech to exclude tongue thrust (figure 6), which can affect production of some sounds (e.g. /s/, /zʹ/, / ʃ/, /dʒ/, /tʃ/and /j/).

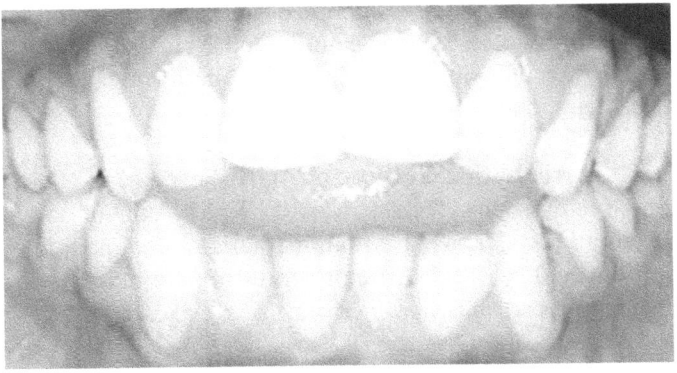

Figure 6: Tongue Thrust
(Source: UtahSpeechTherapy.com)

3. Hearing Screening

If not completed during the speech sound screening, a hearing screening is conducted during the comprehensive speech sound assessment. The screening typically includes otoscopic inspection of the ear, pure tone audiometry and immittance testing.

4. Speech Sound Assessment

The speech sound assessment includes both standardised assessments, e.g. single-word testing and a non-standardised assessment, e.g. connected speech sampling. Articulation and phonological abilities of the child should be assessed by either single word test or connected sample speech or both to identify speech sound errors and phonological patterns. In addition, severity, intelligibility and perception of speech sound should be assessed.

▪ The Articulation Assessment

The articulation assessment examines a child's ability to produce individual speech sounds, either in isolation or in words, by establishing the child's phonetic inventory. The assessment consists of two parts:

- **Articulation ability testing:** The child is asked to name pictures for certain words. Words contain sounds elicited all consonants at initial, medial and final positions in addition to all vowels. Articulation errors are classified into consonant errors and vowel errors.

  A- *Consonant errors:* Substitutions or distortions of certain sounds in all their positions in the word and in all contexts.
  B- *Vowel errors:* Vowel errors (also considered unusual) may also be indicative of abnormal speech development (Pollack, 1991) and include diphthongisation (the splitting apart of the target vowel into two vowel sounds), vowel harmony (when vowels are produced like contrastive vowels elsewhere in a word) and feature changes in terms of tongue placement: backing (tongue retracted for a front vowel, e.g. kite for cat) and fronting (tongue forward for a back vowel, e.g. rake for rack).

- **Speech-sound stimulability:** This task evaluates the ability to imitate the production of an errored consonant in CV/VC syllable context or in isolation. If a child fails to produce a consonant correctly in a word, the examiner asks the child to imitate it in a syllable (allowing three attempts) and then in isolation (Dodd, 2013). Stimulability testing examines the child's ability to imitate a misarticulated sound correctly when a model is provided by the clinician. It provides information about how well the individual imitates the sound in one or more contexts (e.g. isolation, syllable, word, phrase) and helps determine the level of cueing necessary to achieve the best production (e.g. auditory model; auditory and visual model; auditory, visual and verbal model; tactile cues). It is used to determine if the sound is likely to be acquired without intervention, select appropriate therapy targets and predict improvement in therapy (ASHA, 2014).

The Phonology Assessment

The phonological ability of the child should be examined by identifying the phonological error patterns used by the child and classifying them with reference to normative data of the phonological error patterns of the age interval of the examined child as normal and unusual error patterns (Dodd, 2013). Concerning normal error patterns, it should be further classified into; age-appropriate error patterns, delayed error patterns, gross included error patterns (multiple numbers of age-appropriate errors than found in the same age interval of children). It should be considered as one criterion of the phonologically disordered child as the child extends the use of the pattern across a greater range of contexts than his peers (Ingram and Ingram, 2001). One of the normalised phonological tests that mentioned this criterion is MATPP (Abou-Elsaad et al., 2018). If that data is not provided, clinicians can use the criterion of 40% of the examined words (Hodson and Paden, 1991); (Lowe, 1996) in the spontaneous speech sample or the error used in 5 different words on a standard test of 50 words (Dodd, 2014).

Severity

Severity is a qualitative judgement made by the clinician that indicates the degree of impact of the SSD on the child's communication in daily activities. (ASHA, 2014). Simply, degrees of SSD can be classified: mild, moderate and severe or profound (Shriberg et al., 1997). However, the severity should be assessed for both aspects of speech disorder (i.e. for articulation errors and phonological error patterns). For articulation errors, Shriberg and Kwiatkowski (1982) proposed a quantitative approach in which the percentage of consonants correct (PCC) is used to determine severity on a continuum from mild to severe. This type of calculation most closely rates with the listener's perceptions of severity. For example, a PCC of 85-100 is considered "mild" while a PCC of less than 50 is considered "severe". This approach has been modified to include a total of 10 such indices including percent vowels correct (Shriberg et al, 1997).

For phonological error patterns, Edwards (1992) devised a metric to reflect the average number of phonological error patterns (phonological processes) that is used per word, called Process Density Index (PDI). This rough measure of phonological disorder severity is calculated by adding the total number of phonological error patterns that occurred for all words in a sample and dividing by the total number of words. The higher the PDI, the more severe the phonological disorder. Caution should be exercised when using PDI as a severity measure because all error patterns are given equal weight or value. For example, a common substitution error pattern of stopping such as t/s, is given the same value as an unusual substitution, such as w/s. clearly, unusual phonological error pattern will negatively impact intelligibility and thus increase the severity of the phonological disorder more so than the common phonological error pattern. The PDI supplements PCC in evaluating severity of SSD and may be more sensitive than the PCC, which only reveals the presence or absence of a correctly produced consonant in a particular word.

Intelligibility

Intelligibility is a subjective perceptual judgement based on how much of the child's spontaneous speech is understood by the listener. Intelligibility can range from "intelligible" (message is completely understood) to "unintelligible" (message is not understood). Intelligibility is a factor that is frequently used when judging the severity of the child's speech problem (Kent et al., 1994). It is often used to decide the need for intervention and to evaluate progress in therapy. A child of 3 years of age or older who is unintelligible is recognised as a candidate for treatment (Bernthal et al., 2013).

A guideline for expected conversational intelligibility levels of typically developing children talking to unfamiliar listeners can be calculated by dividing the child's age in years by 4 and converting that number into a percentage:1 year— 25% intelligible; 2 years—50% intelligible; 3years—75% intelligible; 4 years—100% intelligible (Flipsen, 2006).

Although the degree of speech intelligibility is a subjective judgement, a number of quantitative measures have been suggested including calculating the percentage of words understood in the speech sample (Bauman-Waengler, 2012). By dividing the number of words that can be understood by the total number of words produced and multiplying by 100, an intelligibility percentage is calculated (Peña-Brooks and Hedge, 2007). There is no single intelligibility assessment procedure that is appropriate for all children across settings and intelligibility may vary depending on the setting.

Several factors can influence the intelligibility of speech, including: level of communication (e.g. single words vs. conversation); listener's familiarity with the speaker's speech pattern; speaker's rate, stress patterns, pauses, voice quality, loudness and fluency; social environment (e.g. familiar vs. unfamiliar conversational partners, one-on-one vs. group conversation); communication cues for listener (e.g. known vs. unknown context); signal-to-noise ratio (e.g. amount of background noise) and listeners (ASHA, 2014).

Inconsistency Assessment

The child's three productions for each word are compared to determine consistency. It should be noted that, the production accuracy is not rated, but the consistency of the child's three productions is measured.

- *Inconsistent phonological disorder*: At least 40% of words produced variably.
- *Consistent phonological disorder*: At least two atypical patterns and an inconsistency score below 40% (ASHA, 2012).

• *Speech Perception Testing*

Speech perception testing is used to determine if a child is able to perceive the difference between the standard production of a phoneme and his own error production. It may be indicated for children who do not use phonemic contrasts to determine if errors are related to a generalised perceptual problem (Bernthal et al., 2013).

A number of different test examples are used to assess speech sound discrimination, including (Locke, 1980):

1. **Auditory Discrimination**: Minimal pairs containing a single phoneme contrast are presented and the child is instructed to say "same" or "different".
2. **Picture Identification**: The child is shown 2-4 pictures representing words with minimal pairs. The clinician says one of these words and the child is asked to point to the correct picture.
3. **Pronunciation Accuracy/Inaccuracy**: Using sounds the child is suspected of having difficulty perceiving, picture targets containing these cards are used as visual cues and the child is asked to judge whether the speaker says the item correctly (e.g.

picture of a ship is shown; speaker says, "ship" or "s_p").

5. Spoken Language Testing

Language testing is included in a comprehensive speech sound assessment because of the high incidence of co-occurring language problems in children with SSD. The assessment begins with a screening of receptive language and expressive language, then a full language battery is performed if indicated by screening results (Shriberg and Austin, 1998).

6. Phonological Processing

Phonological processing is the use of the sounds of one's language to process spoken and written language. The broad category of phonological processing includes phonological awareness, phonological working memory and phonological retrieval. All three components of phonological processing are important for speech production and the development of spoken and written language skills. It is important to screen phonological processing skills to decide if they should be included in the comprehensive SSD assessment. In addition, it is necessary to monitor the spoken and written language development of children with phonological processing difficulties (ASHA, 2014).

- *Phonological Awareness*: It is the awareness of the sound structure of a language and the ability to consciously analyse and manipulate this structure via a range of tasks, such as phoneme segmentation and blending at the word, onset-rime, syllable and phonemic levels.
- *Phonological Working Memory*: Includes storing phoneme information in a temporary short-term memory. This phonemic information is then readily available for manipulation during phonological awareness tasks. Non-word repetition (e.g. repeat

/pæg/) is one example of a phonological working memory task.

- *Phonological Retrieval*: It is the ability to recall the phonemes associated with specific graphemes, which can be assessed by rapid naming tasks (e.g. rapid naming of letters and numbers). This ability to recall the speech sounds in one's language is also integral to phonological awareness.

7. Literacy Assessment [Reading and Writing]

Difficulties with the speech processing system (e.g. listening, discriminating, remembering and producing speech sounds) can lead to both speech production and phonological awareness difficulties that can hinder the development of literacy (Anthony et al., 2011). Children who perform well on sound awareness tasks become successful readers and writers, while children who struggle with such tasks often do not. In their "critical age" hypothesis, Bishop and Adams (1990) stated that children who are not intelligible by 5½ years of age will likely have difficulties with decoding and spelling.

Components of the *literacy assessment* include the following depending on the child's age and expected stage of literacy development (ASHA, 2014):

1. *Print Awareness* (recognising that books have a front and back and that the direction of words is from left to right and recognising where words on the page start and stop).
2. *Alphabet Knowledge* (including naming/printing alphabetic letters from A to Z).
3. *Phoneme-Grapheme Correspondence* (knowing that letters have sounds and knowing the sounds for corresponding letters and letter combinations).
4. *Reading Decoding* (using phoneme-grapheme knowledge to segment and blend sounds in grade-level words).

5. *Spelling* (using phoneme-grapheme knowledge to spell grade-level words).
6. *Reading Fluency* (reading smoothly without frequent or significant pausing).
7. *Reading Comprehension* (understanding grade-level text, including the ability to make inferences).

Classification of speech disorder: a diagnostic summary chart

Name: Age: (y:m)   Date tested:

What are the characteristics of the child's speech?

Articulation of phones

Consonants						Vowels and diphthongs		Suprasegmental	
I	F		F	I	F	i	eı	Quality	
p		θ		w		ı	ə	Pitch	
b		ð		h		ɛ	oʊ	Loudness	
t		s		Extra phones		æ	aı	Flexibility	
d		z				ʌ	aʊ	Intonation	
k		ʃ				a	ɔı	Rate	
g		ʒ				ɒ	ıə	
m		r				ɔ	ɔə	
n		tʃ				ʊ	ʊə	
ŋ		dʒ				u	ɛə	
f		l				ə		
v		j						

Phonological error patterns

Developmental	Non-developmental	Syllable structures	
assimilation	initial-cons. Deletion	CV	CCVCC
cluster reduction:	medial-cons. Deletion	VC	CCCV
/s/ + C	Backing	CVC	VCCC
C + lrw j	Glottalization	CCV	CCCVC
nasal + C	intrusive cons.	VCC	CVCCC
weak-syll. deletion	uses non-native phones	Additional error patterns	
final-cons. deletion	assimilation across words		
stopping	uses favourite sound		
fronting	Consistency Index		
voicing	Percentage of words produced inconsistently: ___ %		
gliding			

Presence of disorder

Articulation	Delay	Consistent Disorder	Inconsistent Disorder
Other (specify)			

How severe is the speech disorder and what are its consequences?

Severity rating	Consequences of disorder	
Percentage phonemes correct:	Behaviour	
Clinician intelligibility rating:	Personality	
Child awareness/concern:	Family relationships	
Caregiver awareness/concern:	Peer relationships	
School awareness/concern:	Academic performance	

Can any causal and maintenance factors be identified?

Organic		Non-organic	
Any impairment of		Concern re:	
• Hearing		• Language-learning environment	
• Auditory processing		• Caregiver communication skills	
• Speech anatomy		• Language stimulation	
• Oro-motor function		• Sibling interference	
• Intellectual function		• Emotional trauma	
• Neurological function		• Family dynamics	
History of:		• School adjustment	
• Genetic predisposition		Specify Other:	
• Significant health problems			
• Delayed milestones			
Specify Other:		Age of onset:	
		• Congenital	
		• Developmental	
		• Acquired	

Initial management decisions

Further assessment of communication?	Referrals for assessment of:
Intervention indicated?	

Figure 7: A Diagnostic Sheet for Diagnosis of Speech Sound Disorder

Source: Dodd, 2013

Special Considerations

❖ *Assessing Young, Unintelligible and/or Reluctant Children*

Young children might not be able to follow directions for standardised tests, might have limited expressive vocabulary and might produce words that are unintelligible. Other children, regardless of age, may produce less intelligible speech or be unwilling to speak in an assessment setting. Strategies for collecting an adequate speech sample with these populations include obtaining a speech sample during the assessment session using play activities, involving parents in the session to encourage talking, asking parents to supplement data from the assessment session by recording the child's speech at home during spontaneous conversation, asking parents to keep a log of the child's intended words and how these are pronounced (ASHA, 2014).

Sometimes, the SSD is so severe that the child's intended message cannot be understood. However, even when a child's speech is unintelligible, it is usually possible to obtain information about his speech sound production. For example a single-word test provides opportunities for production of recognisable units of sound and these productions can usually be transcribed; it may be possible to understand and transcribe a spontaneous speech sample by using a structured situation to provide context when obtaining the sample, commenting the recorded sample by repeating the child's utterances, when possible, to facilitate later transcription (ASHA, 2014).

❖ *Assessing Bilingual/Multilingual Populations*

Assessment of a bilingual individual requires an understanding of both linguistic systems, because the sound system of one language can affect the sound system of the other language. The assessment process must identify whether differences are truly related to SSD or are normal variations of speech caused by the first language. When assessing a bilingual or multilingual individual, clinicians gather information, including language history and language use to determine which language(s) should be assessed; phonemic inventory, phonological structure and syllable structure of the other language; dialect of the individual; assess phonological skills in both languages in single words as well as in spontaneous speech sample; determine if difficulty in discriminating phonemes in one language is due to the presence of these sounds as allophones in the child's primary language and detect the child's normal error patterns, unusual error patterns and cross linguistic effects (Fabiano-Smith and Goldstein, 2010).

Prognosis of SSD

In addition to the age of the child, the type of disorder, severity of the disorder, family support and child motivation, there are some of the many prognostic indicators clinicians should take into consideration (Stein-Rubin and Fabus, 2011).

1. **Consistency of phonetic errors**: The more consistent the error, the less likely the child will be stimulable in therapy or spontaneously remediate the error production.
2. **Stimulability**: This reflects a child's ability to correctly imitate a given sound when provided with specific instructions and models of the sound and stimulable sounds can be remediated easily.
3. **External error sound discrimination:** (the auditory ability to differentiate the sound from other sounds when presented): Decreased ability to discriminate a target sound error from other productions is a poor prognostic indicator.
4. **Internal error sound discrimination**: (ability to self-evaluate production of target sound from incorrect production): Decreased internal error sound discrimination is a poor prognostic indicator.

5. **Unusual phonological error patterns**: Such as backing, initial consonant deletion, nasal preference (substitution of /n/ and /m/ for stops and fricatives) and tetism (substitution of /t/ for /f/). These unusual patterns are red flags for poor prognosis. Vowel errors (also considered unusual) may also be indicative of abnormal speech development.

6. **Co-morbid factors**: These can affect speech-language acquisition and include hearing impairment, attention deficit hyperactive disorder, autistic spectrum disorder, intellectual disability and brain damaged motor handicapped (BDMH) disease and learning disorders.

The use of speech sound assessment procedures can be done for children with speech sound disorders either due to organic causes or functional. After complete and careful assessment, clinicians can determine the cause of the SSD, the articulation errors, stimulability, phonological error patterns, severity, intelligibility, speech perception, comorbid disorders and prognosis, thus they can reach the diagnosis of a subtype of SSD and choose the appropriate therapy plan that lead to good improvement in a short time.

Treatment of SSD depends on its subtypes e.g. treatment of articulation disorders focuses on speech correction, helping children to improve their articulation by remediation of one sound at a time, while treatment of phonological disorders focuses on building and reorganising children's phonological representations rather than improving the surface articulation of speech sounds (Justice, 2006).

Chapter Summary

This chapter defines speech sound disorders, describes their aetiology, diagnostic criteria and their subtypes in addition to a comprehensive approach to their diagnosis and finally, the prognosis.

References

Abou-Elsaad, T., Afsah, O., & Rabea, M. (2018). Identification of Phonological Processes in Arabic–Speaking Egyptian Children by Single-word Test. Journal of communication disorders.

American Speech – Language – Hearing Association. (2014): Speech Sound Disorders: Articulation and Phonological Processes. American Speech Language Hearing Association. Retrieved 17, March, 2014 from http://www.asha.org/public/speech/disorders/speechsounddisorders.htm.

American Speech-Language-Hearing Association. (2012): Speech Sound Disorders.Retrievedfrom http://csd.wp.uncg.edu/wp-content/uploads/sites /6/2012/12/ DPI_Speech_Sound _Disorders 9.261.pdf.

Anthony, J. L., Aghara, R. G., Dunkelberger, M. J., Anthony, T. I., Williams, J. M., and Zhang, Z. (2011): What factors place children with speech sound disorders at risk for reading problems? American Journal of Speech-Language Pathology, 20(2), 146-160.

Bankson, N. W., Bernthal, J. E., & Flipsen, P. (2009). Phonological assessment procedures. In J. E. Bernthal, N. W. Bankson & P. Flipsen (Eds.), Articulation and phonological disorders: Speech sound disorders in children (pp. 187-250). Boston: Pearson.

Bauman-Waengler, J. (2012): Articulatory and phonological impairments: A clinical focus (4th Ed.). Pearson Higher Ed.

Berntha., J. E., Bankson, N. W., and Flipsen, P. (2013): Articulation and phonological disorders: Speech sound disorders in children (7th ed.). Upper Saddle River, NJ: Pearson.

Bishop, D., and Adams, C. (1990): A prospective study of the relationship between specific language impairment, phonological disorders, and reading retardation. Journa. of Child Psychology and Psychiatry, 31, 1027-1050.

Bowen, C. (2015). Five levels of speech function with examples of difficulties that might occur at each level. Retrieved 31 December 2016,fromwww.speechlanguagetherapy.com/index.php?option=com_content&view=article&id=45:cl assification&catid=11:admin&Iemid=121.

Dinnsen. D. A., and Charles-Luce, J. (1984): Phonological neutralization, phonetic implementation and individual differences. Journal of Phonetics, 12(1), 49-60.

Dodd, B., 2011: Differentiating speech delay from disorder. Does it matter? Topics in Language Disorders, 31(2), 96–111.

Dodd, B. (2013). Differential diagnosis and treatment of children with speech disorder. John Wiley & Sons.

Dodd, B. (2014): Differential Diagnosis of Pediatric Speech Sound Disorder. Current Developmental Disorders Reports, 1(3), 189-196.

Eadie, P., Morgan, A., Ukoumunne, O. C., Ttofari Eecen, K., Wake, M. and Reilly, S. (2015): Speech sound disorder at 4 years: prevalence, comorbidities, and predictors in a community cohort of children. Developmental Medicine & Child Neurology, 57: 578–584. doi: 10.1111/dmcn.12635.

Edwards, M. L. (1992): In support of phonological processes. Language, Speech, and Hearing Services in Schools, 23(3), 233-240.

Edwards, M. L., and Shriberg, L. D. (1983): Phonology: Applications in communicative disorders. College Hill Press.

Fabiano, Leah and Goldstein, Brian (2010): Early-, Middle-, and Late-Developing Sounds in Monolingual and Bilingual Children: An Exploratory Investigation. American Journal of Speech-Language Pathology. Vol.19, 66-77.

Flipsen, P., Jr. (2006): Measuring the intelligibility of conversational speech in children. Clinical Linguistics and Phonetics, 20(4), 202-312.

Freiberg, C., Wicklund, A., and Squier, S. (2003): Speech and language impairments assessment and decision making technical assistance guide. Madison, WI: Wisconsin Department of Public Instruction.

Grunwell, P. (1985): Phonological Assessment of Child Speech (PACS). Windsor, Berks: NFER-Nelson.

Hodson, B. W., and Paden, E. P. (1991). A phonological approach to remediation: Targeting intelligible speech. Austin, TX: Pro Ed.

Ingram, D., and Ingram, K. D. (2001): A whole-word approach to phonological analysis and intervention. Language, speech, and hearing services in schools, 32(4), 271-283.

Kent, R. D., Miolo, G., and Bloedel, S. (1994): The intelligibility of children's speech: A review of evaluation procedures. American Journal of Speech-Language Pathology, 3, 81-95.

Leitão, S. (2011): My top 10 assessment resources (with a pediatric slant). ACQuiring Knowledge in Speech, Language and Hearing, 13, 94–95.

Lewis, B. A., Shriberg, L. D., Freebairn, L. A., Hansen, A. J., Stein, C. M., Taylor, H. G., & Iyengar, S. K. (2006). The genetic bases of speech sound disorders: Evidence from spoken and written language. Journal of Speech, Language, and Hearing Research, 49(6), 1294-1312.

Locke, J. (1980): The inference of speech perception in the phonologically disordered child. Part I: A rationale, some criteria, the conventional tests. Journal of Speech and Hearing Disorders, 45, 431-444.

Lowe, R. J. (1996): Assessment link between phonology and articulation: ALPHA (rev. ed.). Mifflinville, PA: Speech and Language Resources.

Peña-Brooks, A., and Hegde, M. N. (2007): Assessment and treatment of articulation and phonological disorders in children (2nd ed.). Austin, TX: Pro-Ed.

Pollack, K. E. (1991): The identification of vowel errors using traditional articulation or phonological process test stimuli. LSHS, 22, 39–50.

Shriberg, L. D., and Austin, D. (1998): Comorbidity of speech-language disorders: Implications for a phenotype marker for speech delay. In R. Paul (Ed.), the speech-language connection (pp. 73-117). Baltimore, MD: Brookes.

Shriberg, L. D., and Kwiatkowski, J. (1982): Phonological disorders II: A conceptual framework for management. Journal of Speech and Hearing Disorders, 47, 242-256.

Shriberg, L. D., Austin, D., Lewis, B., McSweeny, J. L., and Wilson, D. L. (1997): The percentage of consonants correct (PCC) metric: Extensions and reliability data. Journal of Speech, Language, and Hearing Research, 40, 708-722.

Stein-Rubin, C., and Fabus, R. (2011). Assessment of articulation and phonological disorders: A Guide to Clinical Assessment and Professional Report Writing in Speech-Language Pathology. Nelson Education.

Williams, A. L. (2000): Multiple oppositions: Theoretical foundations for an alternative contrastive intervention approach. American Journal of Speech-Language Pathology, 9, 282-288.